The Doctor's Perspective

A LOOK AT TESTOSTERONE, WELLNESS AND PERFORMANCE

Dr. Khashayar Farzam

Copyright © 2025 by Khashayar Farzam

All rights reserved.

No portion of this book may be reproduced in any form without written permission from the author.

ISBN: 978-1-0691997-0-6

Independently published

Disclaimer: This book is intended solely for educational purposes and reflects the author's personal opinion only. The content herein is not medical advice and should not be construed as such. Readers are strongly advised to consult with a qualified healthcare professional before making any decisions regarding medical treatments, supplements, or lifestyle changes discussed in this book. The information provided is based on research and clinical experience, but it may not apply to every individual's specific circumstance or medical history.

The author assumes no responsibility for any consequences arising from the use or misuse of the information presented. All medical decisions should strictly be made in consultation with a licensed healthcare provider who understands your unique health needs. The views expressed in this book do not represent the policies or opinions of any medical institution or organization.

Book Cover by Olivia Pro Design

Copy editing by Karine Farzam

For correspondence, including questions, concerns, or errata, please contact: info@doctorfarzam.com or visit www.doctorfarzam.com

Table of Contents

Legal Disclaimer..1

Chapter 1: Introduction..3
An overview of the book's themes: testosterone, PEDs, and wellness. Defining evidence-based medicine vs. anecdotal evidence and the importance of informed decisions.

Chapter 2: Science vs. Broscience......................................5
Exploring the origins of "broscience," its characteristics, and how it contrasts with peer-reviewed research. Identifying common myths and misinformation in fitness and wellness.

Chapter 3: Exploring Online Discourse: The World of TRT, Anabolic Steroids, Supplements, and Misconceptions...............9
A historical perspective on the rise of online communities, the spread of dogmatic teachings, and the evolving narrative around TRT and anabolic steroids.

Chapter 4: Introducing the Pillars of Men's Health................15
A holistic review of testosterone's role in health, including its relationship with cardiac and prostate health, hypogonadism, and obesity.

Chapter 5: A Closer Look at Hypogonadism........................19
Understanding low testosterone, its causes, symptoms, and the importance of diagnosis and management.

Chapter 6: Testosterone Replacement Therapy....................29
An in-depth look at TRT, its benefits, risks, methods of administration, and the need for careful monitoring and lifestyle considerations.

Chapter 7: Clomid, SERMS, and HCG................................49
Going beyond TRT, this chapter explores alternative treatment options for hypogonadism.

Chapter 8: Understanding Gynecomastia..........................55
A look at one of the potential side effects of exogenous androgen use.

Chapter 9: Acne – A Common Side Effect: A Review of Treatment Methods..59
Acne has had a long-standing association with hormonal changes. This chapter looks at what acne is and how it can be managed.

Chapter 10: Access to Testosterone Replacement Therapy and Lifestyle Monitoring..65
A look at why TRT can be hard to access for some, and why it may not be the answer for everyone.

Chapter 11: A Look at Guidelines: What do Medical Societies Around the World Think about TRT?..69
The medical literature and guidelines are both consistent and inconsistent around the world depending on the context. This chapter reviews various nations' TRT guidelines.

Chapter 12: Erectile Dysfunction – When Testosterone is Not Enough...75
As a common symptom of hypogonadism, erectile dysfunction is still its own entity. This chapter looks at other causes and various treatments.

Chapter 13: An Introduction to Anabolic Steroids and Performance Enhancing Drugs...85
Looking at anabolic steroids and PEDs. Analysis of their effects, common usage patterns, and associated risks.

Chapter 14: Major Injectable Anabolic Steroids.....................89
A look at a very broad range of injectable steroids

Chapter 15: Major Oral Anabolic Steroids.........................101
Oral steroids can pose unique health risks, this chapter reviews oral anabolic steroids.

Chapter 16: Prohormones..111
Detailed look at various prodrugs that convert to active anabolic steroids inside the body.

Chapter 17: Steroids in the Clinical Setting: A Closer Look at Side Effects, Preventative Care, Medical Treatment and Common Lab Findings..117
This chapter provides an outline for healthcare professionals and curious patients on the nuanced medical approach to anabolic steroids.

Chapter 18: Drug Use in Sports...131
The history and ethics of performance enhancing drug use in competitive sports, with a focus on health consequences and the impact on sportsmanship.

Chapter 19: Performance-Enhancing Drugs.......................135
Overview of performance enhancing drugs such as SARMs, peptides, insulin, and EPO, as well as their mechanisms, health implications, and ethical considerations.

Chapter 20: Supplements..157
Evidence-based reviews of common supplements, including protein powders, testosterone boosters, and nootropics, with an emphasis on their safety and efficacy.

Chapter 21: A Closer Look at Creatine..............................175
A deep dive into one of the most common supplements.

Chapter 22: Androgenic Alopecia......................................179
Hormonal causes of hair loss, the role of DHT, and treatment options like finasteride and advanced interventions.

Chapter 23: Prostate Health: The Case for Prostate Cancer Screening..187
Examining prostate-related conditions and the evidence around testosterone's impact on prostate cancer risks.

Chapter 24: Comprehensive Overview of Cardiac Health and Lipid Management..193
Insight into cardiovascular health and various risk factors.

Chapter 25: Metabolic Syndrome: Understanding the Epidemic of Modern Times..209
Metabolic syndrome is a major contributor to many illnesses in the modern era. This chapter explores what it is and how it can be prevented.

Chapter 26: Obesity and Treatment Options........................215
Interlinking obesity, hormonal health, and chronic diseases with strategies for effective management.

Chapter 27: Fatty Liver Disease: Diagnostics and Treatment Options...223
Now called, metabolic dysfunction-associated steatotic liver disease (MASLD), this illness affects one-third of those in Western countries.

Chapter 28: Nutrition: Macros, Myths and A Review of Popular Diets..229
Debunking nutrition myths, macronutrient essentials, and a thorough look at popular diets.

Chapter 29: Building Muscle and Protein - What's the Scoop?..243
Protein intake has been a controversial topic for many years. Just how much do you actually need?

Chapter 30: A Review of Important Studies........................249
A critical analysis of key studies on testosterone, TRT, PEDs, and their implications for men's health and wellness.

Chapter 31: Conclusion..261
Summarizing the evidence-based approach to testosterone, wellness, and PED use while emphasizing individualized health choices.

References..265

Legal Disclaimer

This book is intended solely for educational purposes and reflects the author's personal opinion only. The content herein is not medical advice and should not be construed as such. Readers are strongly advised to consult with a qualified healthcare professional before making any decisions regarding medical treatments, supplements, or lifestyle changes discussed in this book. The information provided is based on research and clinical experience, but it may not apply to every individual's specific circumstance or medical history.

The author and publisher assume no responsibility for any consequences arising from the use or misuse of the information presented. All medical decisions should strictly be made in consultation with a licensed healthcare provider who understands your unique health needs. The views expressed in this book do not represent the policies or opinions of any medical institution or organization.

Chapter 1: Introduction

Testosterone, performance-enhancing drugs (PEDs), and wellness are topics that sit at the crossroads of health, fitness, and controversy. They spark endless debates in gyms, clinics, and online forums, where science often collides with both good and bad anecdotes. This book seeks to bridge the gap between evidence-based medicine and the real-world experiences that dominate these conversations. Whether you are a healthcare professional, a fitness enthusiast, or someone exploring these topics for personal reasons, the goal here is to provide clarity in an area often clouded by misinformation. The focus is not just on the biological and pharmacological aspects, but also on the human element—what drives people to seek solutions, and what outcomes they can realistically expect.

The modern fitness and health landscape is saturated with conflicting advice. Message boards, social media, Facebook groups and YouTube videos have become the go-to resources for many, offering a mix of valuable and accurate information but also harmful misconceptions. This phenomenon sometimes simplifies complex topics such as testosterone replacement therapy (TRT), anabolic steroids, workout advice, and nutrition into anecdotal experience-based advice. While some of this information holds merit, a lot of it lacks the depth and nuance provided by high quality scientific studies. This book explores these myths and contrasts them with peer-reviewed research and clinical expertise, emphasizing the importance of critical thinking and evidence-based practice in navigating the ever-evolving world of health and wellness.

A key element in this exploration is testosterone, a hormone that is essential for physical, mental, and sexual health in men. From its role in athletic performance to its medical application in treating hypogonadism, testosterone has become a focal point in discussions about male health. Yet, it is also misunderstood, with many viewing it as either a miracle drug or some sort of danger. By examining testosterone's physiological roles, its use in therapies like TRT, and its misuse in sports and bodybuilding, this book provides a comprehensive view of its benefits and risks. It also goes into related topics such as hair loss, obesity, cardiac health, and prostate health, showing how they intertwine with hormonal balance and overall wellness.

Ultimately, this book is not about dictating a one-size-fits-all solution but rather to provide the tools to make informed decisions. The chapters ahead will blend scientific rigor with practical insight. Whether you are seeking performance optimization, health related guidance, or simply a better understanding of these complex topics, the aim is to help you achieve a balanced, evidence-based perspective. Wellness is about more than hormones or supplements; it is about integrating knowledge, lifestyle, and personal context to create sustainable health.

Finally, if you are a doctor looking to learn more about these topics for your patients, then you have found the right book.

Chapter 2: Science vs. Broscience

"Broscience" is a colloquial term which is usually used to describe pseudoscience in the context of fitness, subtypes of wellness, bodybuilding, supplements, nutrition, TRT and of course anabolic steroids. It is usually shared by non-experts or enthusiasts who rely on anecdotal evidence and personal experience instead of evidence-based data. The term highlights advice that may sound logical or convincing but lacks empirical backing. Although, it is important to be mindful of the fact that a lot of online advice is accurate; it is simply a matter of sorting out what is and is not legitimate.

Why does it matter? The fitness world has for a long time been entrenched with a large mixture of information that ranges from evidence-based to nonsensical and everything in between. Much of online advice was found on various anonymous message boards in the 2000s and for most of the 2010s. In the 2020s, these fitness enthusiasts have turned to Facebook groups and reddit as their primary source of information and discussion. Unfortunately, there has not been a methodology to truly differentiate what advice stems from an evidence-based point of view versus what is simply one person's experience. Regardless of your goals, you want credible sources of information that discuss facts. Otherwise, a lot of time can be wasted following advice that yields no results or even causes harm.

Key characteristics to help identify "broscience" information:

- **Anecdotal Evidence**: Usually based on personal stories or gym folklore, with claims such as, "It worked for me, so it will work for you." People are all different and while some anecdotal evidence can be legitimate, not everyone has the same results when doing something.
- **Unscientific Claims**: Ideas that sound scientific but have little to no backing from research or clinical trials. For example, "You need to eat every two hours to 'keep your metabolism running.'"

- **Over-simplified Advice**: It tends to reduce complex biological processes into easy-to-digest tips, which can mislead people into thinking there is a one-size-fits-all approach to fitness.
- **Citing fringe data:** It is not unusual to find studies and data that back up just about any claim. Therefore, it is also not uncommon to find isolated studies that can back up fringe claims. Critical analysis of the study and its methodology, and a look at the total body of evidence is important to differentiate this.

Common examples of "broscience":

- *"You need to eat protein immediately after your workout or your workout will be wasted."*
- *"Carbs at night turn directly into fat."*
- *"Doing high reps will make you more 'toned.'"*
- *"You need protein every 2-3 hours or you will become catabolic"*

While these types of tips might have some truth or be loosely based on real science, they are often over-exaggerated or misinterpreted. It is best to rely on peer-reviewed research that has cumulative evidence. If that is not possible due to lack of availability, then legitimate expert opinion can also be used. The difference here is that expert opinion is based off from the experience of numerous cases rather than relying on the anecdotal experience of one individual.

Science is grounded in evidence-based research, relying on the scientific method to gather data, test hypotheses, and reach conclusions. It involves rigorous peer review, replication of experiments, and the use of controlled studies to validate findings. Scientific knowledge is continually updated as new evidence emerges, and it aims to minimize bias through structured methodologies. In the context of fitness, nutrition, or medicine, science relies on clinical trials, biochemical research, and long-term studies to provide accurate information that can be applied to various populations.

Online advice is often anecdotal and lacks the structured, methodical approach of science. That is of course not to say that this is true for all general online advice. There is now an abundance of quality information available as well; information which is accurate and scientific. Learning to identify when the information being shared deviates from an evidence-based approach and focuses on personal opinions and experiences has become a new hurdle in improving one's health and wellness.

Chapter 3: Exploring Online Discourse: The World of TRT, Anabolic Steroids, Supplements, and Misconceptions

This chapter will explore the online discourse surrounding anabolic steroids, testosterone replacement therapy (TRT) as well as the use of supplements for fitness. These topics will be discussed individually in significantly greater detail in later chapters.

Anabolic steroids

Anabolic steroid use became quite widespread in the 1980s. Before the age of the internet, steroid users would take whatever was available through their gym friends or even their coach. This would often lead to steroid cycles that would consist of more than one oral compound or various injectable compounds, with or without testosterone. While the end results of gaining muscle mass and strength were well known, the adverse effects were poorly understood; a common example being the hypothalamic pituitary adrenal (HPA) axis suppression of natural testosterone. It was not until the 2000s that the internet helped circulate more information on these issues. To some extent, this was an example of online platforms being successful in circulating some accurate information on this topic.

In the 2000s and 2010s, various online message boards became digital guides for using steroids. It was how users learned about various steroids, their side effects, how to use them, and even what they should do after using them. Recommended regimens were developed and numerous dogmatic teachings spread; however, much of this information was based solely on anecdotal data. While there was indeed a lot of accurate information available, many dogmatic principles lacking scientific evidence were also integrated into the content.

The entire world of online advice played a significant role in the misuse of anabolic steroids, especially in the bodybuilding and fitness communities, where variable advice often circulated freely. This usually led to widespread misconceptions about dosage, cycles, and the potential benefits and risks of anabolic steroid use. Luckily, some scientifically accurate information also circulated on numerous message boards and still does to this day; this information helped minimize harm and guided users to making safer choices. However, those who were not well versed in this area could struggle to identify this accurate information hidden amidst anecdotal information. Admittedly, many steroid users are quite educated on the adverse effects of steroids and many would dig deeper to find out the truth.

With the help of these online communities, users began designing steroid cycles with various compositions. After finishing a steroid cycle, users were urged by their peers to complete a post-cycle therapy (PCT) which typically consisted of using breast cancer medication to reverse the shutdown of endogenous testosterone production. While there was never any evidence shown in scientific literature that PCT is effective or safe, the proposed mechanisms were reasonable in theory.

Over the years, there was an evolution online on the type of advice given and the information that was presented. The use of "PCT" was not necessarily as popular going through the 2010s and later 2020s. As well, the use of mid-cycle aromatase inhibitors had variable popularity. Again, none of these interventions had any clinical evidence backing them up. Much of that, was simply due to the fact that this area of healthcare has not been well studied to date. Many recreational users would simply "cycle off" anabolic steroids and do nothing else, whereas some users utilized numerous other agents simultaneously. Everyone had anecdotal results across the spectrum and their personal experience was shared with others.

Testosterone Replacement Therapy
In the realm of testosterone replacement therapy (TRT), anecdotal information has often distorted the purpose and proper administration of this medical treatment. TRT is designed for men with clinically low testosterone levels, which is diagnosed through a series of blood tests. However, there has been a growing belief that any and all individuals

can directly benefit from testosterone supplementation. In addition, there has been a growing number of men who use the term TRT synonymously with low dose testosterone supplementation. While there is no doubt that supplementation can do wonders for men with low testosterone, there is a different case to be made for those who have normal or even high-normal levels to begin with. Many men, swayed by claims of increased vitality and enhanced physical performance, seek testosterone supplementation without fully understanding its risks. Due to the availability of testosterone through others at their local gym, some men will start low dose testosterone supplementation without undergoing a proper diagnostic evaluation. For men with clinically low testosterone levels, foregoing this investigative step could mean never discovering the underlying cause of their low testosterone. In other cases, individuals may have contraindications that are not discovered until the appropriate workup is done. This is not to say that they will not observe obvious significant performance enhancing effects from exogenous testosterone; but there needs to be due diligence before starting any therapy, especially exogenous hormones.

There can also be misconceptions about TRT dosing and monitoring, specifically for men who do have low testosterone. Instead of following a medically supervised regimen, some individuals self-administer testosterone based on advice from online communities or bodybuilding "gurus". Sometimes this can lead to desirable results. Other times it can result in excessive dosages that push testosterone levels far beyond normal physiological ranges, increasing the risk of side effects such as dyslipidemia or cardiovascular issues. Many of the traditionally reported side effects of testosterone tend to occur at supraphysiologic levels and not physiological levels.

Supplements

The misconceptions discussed above also extend into the world of supplements. A lot of the conversation around supplements is dominated by unproven or exaggerated claims about various products. Protein powders, pre-workouts, fat burners, and testosterone boosters are often marketed as miracle solutions for building muscle, losing fat, or increasing strength, despite many of these claims lacking scientific support. This issue was far more prominent in the 2000s as supplements were sold with exaggerated marketing claims. Nowadays, most users tend to have a better grasp on what they can expect from supplements. To some extent, this can be credited to various online communities, again highlighting that there is good information available.

Advice in some of these communities tends to focus on anecdotal experiences, promoting the idea that taking large amounts of these supplements will lead to faster results, regardless of individual dietary needs, metabolism, or underlying health conditions. While many of these supplements do in fact have evidence-based sources that support their use, online claims can go beyond the scientific parameters.

Testosterone-boosting supplements were an area where consumers often got misled, though less so today. Many of these products are marketed as "natural" alternatives to TRT, claiming to significantly increase testosterone levels, muscle mass, libido, and energy. While certain ingredients like zinc and vitamin D may support healthy testosterone levels, most over-the-counter testosterone boosters lack scientific evidence to back their claims. Additionally, for men with clinically low testosterone, these supplements rarely have a meaningful impact compared to medically prescribed therapies like TRT. It is for that reason that TRT is the recommended treatment for men with low testosterone, rather than using supplements.

The concept of nutrient timing is another area heavily influenced by unproven claims. A popular belief used to be that consuming protein immediately after a workout is critical for muscle growth, with the notion that there is a "magic window" of 30 minutes when muscles are most receptive to protein and stimulating muscle growth. While consuming protein post-workout is beneficial, the evidence has shown that total daily protein intake is far more important than the exact timing of the intake. Overemphasis on nutrient timing can cause individuals to fixate on one variable rather than the big picture. Also, adding strict rules to a regime can lead to burnout and loss of interest over time.

This focus on timing also extends to other supplements, such as creatine or branched-chain amino acids (BCAAs). Advice often suggests that these supplements must be taken at specific times to be effective, even though research indicates that timing is usually less important than consistency.

Perhaps the most significant impact of exaggerated claims about supplements is the overemphasis on their importance. In many fitness circles, people are led to believe that supplements are essential for achieving their goals, causing them to focus more on powders and pills than on foundational factors like a balanced diet, good training, consistency, and proper rest. This overreliance can take away from healthy habits; healthy habits which, in the long run, can be much more productive in achieving one's goals. While some supplements do have evidence supporting their claims and are indeed beneficial, their use should be considered on a case-by-case basis. It is also important to note that some supplements, like creatine, do have evidence backing their efficacy; other supplements may not have any evidence at all. These supplements will circulate through the market over time and eventually fall out of favour for various reasons.

The widespread influence of unverified information on anabolic steroid use, TRT, and supplement practices demonstrates the risks of relying on anecdotal advice on health and fitness. While some advice might offer short-term benefits, it often ignores long-term health consequences and the complexities of individual biology. Myths and oversimplifications can encourage harmful behaviors and mislead individuals into making choices that compromise their well-being. To avoid these pitfalls, it is essential to rely on evidence-based information and be a healthy skeptic.

Chapter 4: Introducing the Pillars of Men's Health

Men's health is a multifaceted area that requires attention to various categories. Traditionally, it focuses on a few topics that are often pertinent to young men, middle aged men and older men. Low testosterone being a common concern as men age is a dominant topic in the world of men's health. Low testosterone can lead to symptoms such as reduced energy, muscle loss, decreased libido, and mood changes. It can also contribute to weight gain, especially in the form of increased abdominal fat. TRT is a potential treatment and can offer great benefits to the right patient. Maintaining a balanced diet, regular exercise, and getting sufficient sleep can also help support healthy testosterone levels naturally, while also improving overall well-being. This highlights why it is critical to ensure all lifestyle factors are appropriately addressed, regardless of TRT use.

Cardiac and prostate health are two major areas of concern for men as they age and are key issues in men's health. Heart disease remains a leading cause of death, with risk factors such as high blood pressure, high cholesterol, obesity, and inactivity. Regular exercise, healthy eating, and managing stress are essential for maintaining a strong cardiovascular system. Prostate health is another critical issue, with conditions such as benign prostatic hyperplasia (BPH) and prostate cancer being more prevalent with age. Additionally, hair loss, often driven by genetic factors and hormonal changes like DHT (dihydrotestosterone) levels, is a common concern that impacts self-esteem among all male age groups; though, is not an issue for some men. Addressing these interconnected health challenges, including obesity, can significantly improve a man's quality of life and longevity.

Low Testosterone: The Silent Disruptor
Testosterone plays a pivotal role in a man's overall health. Produced primarily in the testes, it is crucial to various physiological functions, including muscle strength, bone density, and libido. However, testosterone levels naturally decline with age, and this reduction can

sometimes lead to significant health issues if it declines below a certain threshold. Low testosterone, or hypogonadism, can manifest through a range of symptoms such as fatigue, reduced muscle mass, diminished libido, and mood swings. It is important to note that not everyone's testosterone will have significant decline with age. Many men maintain relatively high testosterone levels into older age whereas many younger men may have low-normal levels. Many men will have no symptoms at all despite having lower levels and others will experience symptoms despite having modestly high levels. There is no definitive rule for this.

The implications of low testosterone extend beyond physical symptoms. Research suggests that this condition can also impact mental health, contributing to depression and diminished cognitive function. Addressing low testosterone involves a multi-faceted approach, including lifestyle changes, medical treatments, and hormone replacement therapy. Recognizing and managing this condition is crucial for maintaining overall health and quality of life. Though, it must be done appropriately and only if the diagnosis is correct. Equally important is to make sure there is no underlying pathologic condition causing the low testosterone due to the numerous implications that come with an endocrine disorder.

Cardiac Health: The Heart of the Matter
Cardiac health is another cornerstone of men's health (and health in general for all), as cardiovascular diseases remain a leading cause of morbidity and mortality worldwide. Men are at higher risk of heart disease as they age. Risk factors such as high blood pressure, high cholesterol, smoking, and sedentary lifestyle contribute significantly to the likelihood of developing heart-related issues.

Understanding and managing cardiac health involves a combination of preventive measures and treatment strategies. Lifestyle modifications, including regular physical activity, a balanced diet, and stress management all play a critical role in reducing cardiovascular risk. Additionally, early detection through regular check-ups and adherence to prescribed treatments are essential for mitigating the effects of heart disease and improving long-term health outcomes. More to come on this later.

Hair Loss: Beyond Vanity
Hair loss is another significant issue affecting many men, with conditions such as androgenetic alopecia (commonly known as male pattern baldness) being particularly prevalent. While often perceived as a cosmetic concern, hair loss can have profound psychological impacts, affecting self-esteem and overall mental health. Though for some it is not an issue.

The causes of hair loss are diverse, including genetic factors, hormonal imbalances, and certain medical conditions. Treatments vary from lifestyle adjustments and topical applications to more advanced and pricey medical interventions such as hair transplant surgery. Addressing hair loss effectively requires a nuanced understanding of its underlying causes and a tailored approach to treatment. It is important to highlight that not every case of hair loss is male pattern baldness; hair loss can be a symptom of an underlying disorder such as autoimmune disease.

Obesity: The Growing Epidemic
Obesity, characterized by excessive body fat that poses health risks, is a pressing issue within men's health. It is linked to numerous chronic conditions, including type 2 diabetes, hypertension, and certain types of cancer. The rising prevalence of obesity is often attributed to modern lifestyle factors, including poor dietary choices, sedentary behavior, and environmental influences. It is often the common denominator of a lot of health problems faced by humans. It is also the primary driver in metabolic disease.

Addressing obesity involves a comprehensive strategy which includes dietary changes, increased physical activity, behavioral modifications, and, in some cases, medical interventions. Understanding the complex interplay of genetic, environmental, and psychological factors is crucial for developing effective strategies to combat obesity and its associated health risks. A lot more on this later.

Chapter 5: A Closer Look at Hypogonadism

What is testosterone?

Testosterone is a hormone primarily produced in the testes in men and in smaller amounts in the ovaries and adrenal glands in women. It plays a crucial role in the development of male characteristics during puberty, such as increased muscle mass, deeper voice, as well as facial and body hair growth. Testosterone also helps regulate sex drive, sperm production, bone density, and red blood cell production. Though commonly associated with men, testosterone is essential for both sexes, contributing to overall health, energy levels, and mood stability. Its levels typically peak during early adulthood and gradually decline with age.

Beyond its role in sexual and physical development, testosterone influences a wide range of bodily functions. It aids in maintaining muscle strength and mass, which is crucial for physical fitness and metabolism. Testosterone also supports cognitive function, mood regulation, and even cardiovascular health. Low levels of testosterone, often referred to as "low T", can lead to fatigue, depression, reduced sexual function, and an increased risk of conditions like osteoporosis. Understanding testosterone's role is vital for recognizing the symptoms of imbalances and ensuring proper treatment when necessary.

How is testosterone made in the body?

Through a few pathways, the body creates testosterone from nothing other than cholesterol. A healthy male can expect to produce up to 7mg daily.

The pathway is shown on the following page:

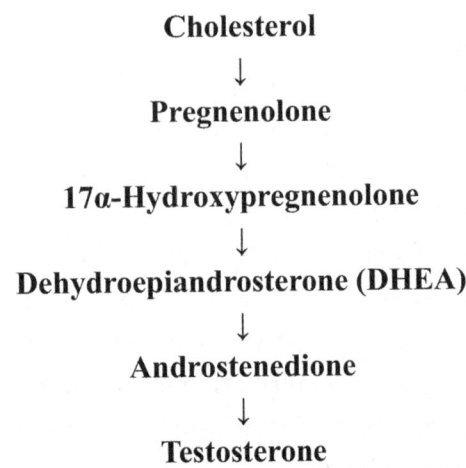

Understanding Low Testosterone (Hypogonadism)
Hypogonadism is a medical condition characterized by the insufficient production of sex hormones, primarily testosterone, in men. As we get older, our testosterone levels may decline. If they decline significantly, it can eventually be categorized as hypogonadism. On the other hand, people of various ages can have low testosterone for numerous reasons.

Hypogonadism can lead to a range of symptoms and health issues, affecting a man's quality of life. This chapter delves into the different types of hypogonadism, their causes, symptoms, diagnosis, and treatment options. Understanding the underlying cause is crucial for ensuring there is no other underlying health problem leading to the low testosterone.

Diagnosing low testosterone is done through blood tests. A few tests are necessary to make the diagnosis and before proceeding into further diagnostic evaluation and treatment.

General lab tests will include:

- **Total testosterone**: This is the sum of all the testosterone in the body and is a key general screening test for low testosterone.

- **Free testosterone:** This is a small fraction of the total testosterone in your body, as almost all testosterone is either bound to sex hormone binding globulin (SHBG) or bound to albumin which is another type of protein. Free testosterone combined with albumin-bound testosterone are what make up the bioavailable testosterone in the body. That is the testosterone that the body is able to actually utilize.
- **Sex hormone binding globulin (SHBG):** This molecule is bound to a large portion of the testosterone in the body. Some conditions that decrease SHBG are obesity or diabetes, whereas aging, for example, can increase it.

Given the variability of levels on a day-to-day basis, the standard of care is to obtain two testosterone level lab tests on different days. To truly optimize accuracy, it should be done fasted between 8-10 AM in the morning. That is when endogenous natural testosterone is at its peak, assuming a normal circadian rhythm is maintained.

Types of Hypogonadism
Hypogonadism is categorized into two primary types: primary and secondary. Understanding these types is important for accurate diagnosis and effective treatment.

Primary Hypogonadism
Primary hypogonadism, also known as primary testicular failure, occurs when the testes themselves are unable to produce sufficient testosterone. This form of hypogonadism is the result of a direct issue with the testes, which can be due to a variety of factors:

Causes of Primary Hypogonadism:
- **Genetic Conditions**: Certain genetic disorders can affect testicular function. For instance, Klinefelter syndrome, a chromosomal abnormality where biological men have an extra X chromosome, can lead to primary hypogonadism. Another condition, Turner syndrome, although typically affecting

biological females, can also lead to primary hypogonadism in males.
- **Injury or Trauma**: Physical injury to the testes, whether from accidents or medical procedures, can impair their ability to produce testosterone. Usually, this would include serious injuries and not minor trauma.
- **Infections**: Mumps virus infection during puberty or adulthood can lead to inflammation and damage of the testes, resulting in decreased testosterone production.
- **Autoimmune Diseases**: In autoimmune conditions, the body's immune system may mistakenly attack the testes, leading to impaired testosterone production. Examples include the following autoimmune polyglandular syndromes (APS):
  - **APS Type 1**: Associated with autoimmune diseases affecting multiple endocrine glands, including hypogonadism due to damage to the gonads.
  - **APS Type 2**: Typically involves adrenal insufficiency, autoimmune thyroid disease, and type 1 diabetes, with hypogonadism as a possible feature.
  - **Autoimmune Orchitis (in males):** The immune system targets the testes, causing inflammation and damage, which can lead to decreased testosterone production and infertility.
  - **Other:** Type 1 diabetes, adrenal insufficiency, Graves disease, and Lupus are all examples of autoimmune diseases that can lead to hypogonadism and low testosterone.

These conditions highlight why it is crucial to undergo a proper evaluation to obtain an accurate diagnosis before starting TRT. Taking testosterone is often necessary in many of these conditions, but the treatment plan may require other components as well.

Diagnosis of Primary Hypogonadism:
Diagnosis involves several steps, including:
- **Medical History and Physical Examination**: A thorough medical history and physical examination help identify symptoms and potential causes of testicular dysfunction. Some

syndromes like Klinefelter syndrome have prominent physical exam findings that help guide the diagnosis. Other things to look out for include small testicles and lack of hair growth. Although, there is some individual variation with these findings. Without this form of assessment, many potential underlying causes can be easily missed.
- **Blood Tests**: Measuring serum testosterone levels is essential and effectively a required step to diagnosing low testosterone. While there will always be controversy over the correct cut off, we can confidently use other biomarkers to differentiate the probable causes of low testosterone. In primary hypogonadism (when the testes themselves do not work properly), testosterone levels are low, but luteinizing hormone (LH) and follicle-stimulating hormone (FSH) levels are elevated due to the body's attempt to stimulate the testes.
- **Genetic Testing**: If a genetic disorder is suspected, karyotyping or other genetic tests may be performed.

Hypothalamus (GnRH)

$\downarrow$

Pituitary Gland (LH & FSH)

$\downarrow$

Testes (Leydig Cells)

$\downarrow$

Testosterone

Treatment Options for Primary Hypogonadism:
- **Testosterone Replacement Therapy**: TRT is the primary treatment for restoring normal testosterone levels. It can be administered through injections, patches, gels, or pellets, though injections are often a preferred method. Other non-testosterone options such as Clomid also exist, with controversial efficacy on

symptom relief. These topics will be explored at length in later chapters.
- **Addressing Underlying Conditions**: If the cause of hypogonadism is a specific condition, such as an infection or autoimmune disorder as mentioned above, treating the underlying condition is incredibly important. While TRT will be started, the underlying condition also needs to be simultaneously treated. An example of this would be someone who has hyperprolactinemia due to a pituitary tumor. This will cause low testosterone, which requires TRT. However, this individual will also require cabergoline to treat the severely high prolactin level and shrink the pituitary tumor.
- **Lifestyle Modifications**: Obesity, poor sleep, sleep apnea, poor diet and other lifestyle habits can lead to low-normal testosterone. Fixing these issues does have a clinically significant and measurable effect on testosterone production in the body. However, true hypogonadism cannot be fixed with lifestyle modifications. While major drops in testosterone levels can occur with severe disturbances in lifestyle (ex. Extreme levels of stress and simultaneous sleep deprivation), these drops are temporary and quickly rebound back to normal. Severely low levels of testosterone are not caused by lifestyle factors.
- **Supplements:** There are no proven supplements that truly increase testosterone to any significant degree. Many supplements, such as those with Zinc or D-aspartic acid, have been around over the years. While there could be marginal benefits, there is no evidence they truly work. Generally, if a deficiency is present, hypogonadism can occur, and it can be resolved with supplementation. For example, while a zinc deficiency is uncommon, it can cause low testosterone.

Secondary Hypogonadism

Secondary hypogonadism, also known as central hypogonadism, occurs due to issues with the hypothalamus or pituitary gland, which are responsible for signaling the testes to produce testosterone. In this type of hypogonadism, the testes work normally but are not receiving adequate stimulation.

Causes of Secondary Hypogonadism:

- **Pituitary Disorders**: Tumors or diseases affecting the pituitary gland, such as prolactinomas or pituitary adenomas, can disrupt hormone signaling, leading to secondary hypogonadism. This is one of the most common causes of secondary hypogonadism.
- **Hypothalamic Disorders**: Conditions affecting the hypothalamus, such as Kallmann syndrome, which impairs the release of gonadotropin-releasing hormone (GnRH), can result in decreased stimulation of the pituitary gland and, consequently, reduced testosterone production.
- **Medications**: Certain medications, such as steroids or opioids, can suppress pituitary function and reduce testosterone levels. Chronic opioid use is a well-known cause of low testosterone as well as alcohol consumption.
- **Chronic Illnesses**: Chronic diseases such as hemochromatosis (iron overload), diabetes, obesity, or HIV can affect the hypothalamic-pituitary-testicular axis, leading to secondary hypogonadism. It is very important to make the correct diagnosis as these illnesses can cause multi-organ disease.

Diagnosis of Secondary Hypogonadism:

- **Medical History and Physical Examination**: Evaluating the patient's medical history and physical symptoms can provide clues to the underlying cause of secondary hypogonadism and help tailor the workup.
- **Blood Tests**: Serum testosterone levels are low in secondary hypogonadism, but unlike primary hypogonadism, LH and FSH levels are low or normal. Further tests, including measurements of pituitary hormones (LH, FSH, and prolactin), are necessary to identify the root cause. Ruling out other secondary causes is also necessary by checking ferritin and

iron levels, hemoglobin A1c, assessment of renal function and liver enzymes and other tests.
- **Imaging Studies**: MRI may be used to visualize the pituitary gland and hypothalamus, identifying any tumors or structural abnormalities. While MRIs are not part of routine physical exams, they can be ordered for patients with certain blood test abnormalities or certain symptoms. If the case remains suspicious, pituitary MRI and testicular ultrasound should be considered regardless of the blood test results. An example of a suspicious case would be someone with very abrupt hypogonadism.

Treatment Options for Secondary Hypogonadism:
- **Addressing the Underlying Cause**: Treating the primary condition affecting the pituitary or hypothalamus can improve testosterone production. For example, treating the pituitary tumor or managing chronic illnesses may restore normal hormonal function, at least to a reasonable extent.
- **Testosterone Replacement Therapy**: Similar to primary hypogonadism, TRT is often used to manage symptoms of low testosterone. However, it is crucial to address the underlying cause simultaneously. This is why it is not the safest approach for the patient to start TRT without ruling out other causes of hypogonadism.

Symptoms of Hypogonadism

The symptoms of hypogonadism can vary depending on the age of onset and the severity of the condition. Common symptoms include:
- **Reduced Libido**: A noticeable decrease in sexual desire and performance. While a reduction in libido is the most common symptom of hypogonadism, there are people with high testosterone who experience low libido and those with high libido who have low-normal testosterone levels. This nuanced topic will be discussed later, as libido is not simply a function of the endocrine system's adequacy.

- **Fatigue**: Persistent tiredness and lack of energy. Although, fatigue can be caused by hundreds of medical conditions.
- **Depression**: Low mood, irritability, and feelings of sadness. Often an underappreciated symptom of low testosterone.
- **Subjective Muscle Weakness**: Decreased muscle mass and strength or difficulty making progress in the gym. It is important to note that hitting a plateau in the gym is very common and does not necessarily equate to low testosterone. Likewise, the term "subjective" is important to highlight as objective muscle weakness is an indicator of myositis (inflammation of the muscles) which is a completely different topic. Patients who experience subjective muscle weakness from low testosterone are very far from the clinical state of muscle weakness.
- **Bone Density Loss**: Increased risk of osteoporosis and fractures. If osteoporosis is diagnosed in a male, then hypogonadism should usually be ruled out as an underlying cause. The risk of osteoporosis is also one reason as to why premature hypogonadism can have negative health impacts.
- **Infertility**: Difficulty conceiving due to impaired sperm production. Often this can be part of a genetic syndrome but could also be due to numerous other causes.
- **Changes in Body Composition**: Increased body fat and decreased muscle mass.
- **Other**: Other implications are currently being studied, but, as of 2024, it is primarily correlative data.

A Closer Look at Libido

This topic deserves more attention since it is the most common symptom of low testosterone. However, less testosterone does not always result in a lower libido and, similarly, higher levels of testosterone do not always result in a high libido; there are people with higher testosterone who have low libido and vice versa. It is important not to have a one-dimensional view on this symptom as it can be affected by multiple factors.

The neurobiology of libido involves a complex interaction between hormones, neurotransmitters, and brain regions that regulate sexual desire. At the core of this process is the hypothalamus, which integrates signals from the body and stimulates the production of gonadotropin-releasing hormone (GnRH), ultimately leading to the release of testosterone in males and estrogen in females—both critical for libido. Dopamine, a key neurotransmitter, plays a significant role in the brain's reward system and is central to initiating sexual motivation, while serotonin can exert an inhibitory effect on sexual desire. Additionally, oxytocin and vasopressin are implicated in sexual arousal and pair bonding, influencing emotional aspects of libido. The limbic system, which includes the amygdala and nucleus accumbens, is also crucial, as it processes emotions and reinforces sexual behaviors. Altogether, these systems interact dynamically to regulate sexual desire, influenced by hormonal states, emotional context, and sensory stimuli. This is why testosterone supplementation on its own does not always fix low libido, though, fortunately, it often does. The takeaway is that the neurobiology of libido goes beyond a simple one-dimensional hormonal process.

Conclusion

Hypogonadism is a significant medical condition that affects men's health and well-being. Understanding the types, causes, symptoms, and treatment options is crucial for effective management. Whether through testosterone replacement therapy, addressing underlying causes, or making lifestyle changes, individuals with hypogonadism can achieve improved quality of life and overall health. Regular follow-up with healthcare professionals and adherence to treatment plans are essential for optimal outcomes.

Chapter 6: Testosterone Replacement Therapy

Introduction to TRT

TRT is a medical treatment designed to address low testosterone levels in men, a condition often referred to as hypogonadism. As discussed in chapter 5, testosterone is a crucial hormone that influences a variety of physiological processes, including muscle mass, bone density, mood regulation, and sexual function. When testosterone levels drop below normal, it can lead to a range of symptoms such as fatigue, reduced libido, and depression. TRT aims to restore testosterone levels to a normal range, thereby alleviating these symptoms and improving overall quality of life.

History of TRT

The history of TRT begins in the late 19th century, when scientists first started exploring the concept of hormones and their role in the body. Early experiments with animal gland extracts were conducted to boost vitality and combat the effects of aging, most notably by Charles-Édouard Brown-Séquard in 1889. He injected himself with a mixture of animal testicle extracts and claimed improvements in energy and physical health, though these effects were later dismissed as placebo. While these early efforts were simplistic and lacked any real scientific rigor, they laid the groundwork for future exploration into hormone therapy.

A major breakthrough was made in the 1930s when scientists first isolated and synthesized testosterone. In 1935, German chemists Adolf Butenandt and Leopold Ruzicka independently succeeded in identifying the hormone and creating synthetic versions, which won Ruzicka a Nobel Prize. This discovery revolutionized the understanding of male hormones and opened the door to more advanced treatments. The first clinical uses of testosterone were soon developed, primarily in the form of injectable testosterone propionate. Early on, TRT was used to treat hypogonadism and related disorders, restoring sexual function and secondary sexual characteristics in men who had deficient hormone levels.

By the mid-20th century, TRT became more established in medical practice, with synthetic forms becoming more refined and widely available. However, the use of TRT remained limited to medical conditions such as hypogonadism or delayed puberty. It was not until the late 20th century and into the early 21st century that TRT gained broader interest for age-related testosterone decline, often referred to as "andropause." As more men began seeking treatment for symptoms associated with aging, such as reduced energy, libido, and muscle mass, testosterone supplementation evolved beyond a treatment for rare medical conditions and entered mainstream discussions about men's health.

Purpose and Benefits of TRT

TRT is primarily used to manage the symptoms of low testosterone levels. This is different than simply taking exogenous testosterone to increase your testosterone to supraphysiologic levels. As the name implies, "replacement" in testosterone *replacement* therapy, means to replace and restore levels to what would be a healthy level. This is a key point to highlight as low dose testosterone, while classified as "TRT dosing" is still not true TRT.

Doctor's Opinion: From a medical point of view, having an optimal level of testosterone is generally healthy and most likely to result in the best symptomatic outcome. However, many patients may have symptoms of low testosterone despite having relatively high natural testosterone. This is where it's important to avoid "anchoring bias" and move onto other explanations for the symptoms rather than just low testosterone.

For healthcare professionals: Deciding to start TRT is both an art and science. While low testosterone levels are a pre-requisite to need TRT, the decision on where to draw the line on what is considered low, is an art. There can be variability in lab ranges, and it is not always fair to say that simply being above the bottom cut-off is truly normal.

TRT's purpose and benefits include:

- **Restoration of Normal Testosterone Levels**: The primary goal of TRT is to bring testosterone levels back to a normal physiological range, which can help alleviate symptoms associated with low testosterone and achieve homeostasis. Our bodies do not respond well to deficiencies of important biochemicals – testosterone is no exception to that.
- **Improvement in Sexual Function**: Low testosterone is often linked to reduced libido and erectile dysfunction. TRT can improve libido and performance by restoring adequate hormone levels. The loss of libido is arguably one of the biggest symptoms of low testosterone and one symptom that can have the most substantial benefit from TRT.
- **Increased Muscle Mass and Strength**: Testosterone plays a significant role in muscle development, as most people know. Patients with low testosterone can experience a decline in muscle mass; this can result in an increased risk of frailty related pathology in the future. TRT can help increase muscle mass and strength, provided that the patient is working out and maintaining a reasonable diet – this lifestyle piece is crucial to maximize the benefits of TRT.
- **Enhanced Bone Density**: Testosterone contributes to bone health. TRT can help prevent bone loss and reduce the risk of osteoporosis. Men with premature osteoporosis should generally be checked for low testosterone.
- **Improved Mood and Cognitive Function**: Many men with low testosterone experience symptoms of depression and anxiety. TRT can enhance mood and day-to-day function by normalizing hormone levels. This does not mean that every case of depression is linked to low testosterone, but it does mean that it can be a consideration. In many cases, low-normal testosterone alongside depression could be a byproduct of certain lifestyle choices.
- **Better Fat Distribution**: Testosterone helps regulate fat metabolism. TRT can assist in reducing abdominal fat and

improving body composition. Again, the lifestyle piece is very important in order to experience this benefit.

Types of TRT

TRT can be administered in several different forms, each with its own set of advantages and considerations. The chosen method will depend on patient preferences, lifestyle, and medical advice. Generally, injectable testosterone is a preferred modality as it allows the most accurate dosing and is the easiest to titrate.

1. Injections

Description: Testosterone injections are one of the most common forms of TRT and perhaps the modality that provides the most accurate method of monitoring and titration. These are intramuscular injections which are performed on a regular basis. Injections can also be performed subcutaneously. Using this method, the hormone is absorbed into the bloodstream, typically in the form of testosterone enanthate or testosterone cypionate.

Benefits:

- **Effective Absorption**: Injections provide a reliable and effective way to increase testosterone levels. It is the easiest modality for dose adjustments.
- **Customizable Dosing**: The dosage and frequency can be tailored to the individual's needs based on their serum levels and symptom relief.

Considerations:

- **Frequency**: Injections are usually given once weekly, if not twice per week, to achieve stable serum levels. While biweekly dosing has been popular in some medical circles, it can lead to large fluctuations.
- **Pain and Discomfort**: Some individuals experience pain or discomfort at the injection site. There is also the risk of infection; although, this can be minimized simply by cleaning the bottle and injection site thoroughly with alcohol pads.

Injectable Testosterone Formulations

Formulation	Brand Name(s)	Dosage	Administration Frequency	Availability (Regions)
Testosterone Enanthate	Delatestryl (USA), Xyosted (USA), Primoteston (Europe)	100 mg per week (can vary)	Weekly	USA, Canada, Europe, Australia
Testosterone Cypionate	Depo-Testosterone (USA), AndroCyp (Australia)	100 mg per week (can vary)	Weekly	USA, Canada, Australia
Testosterone Propionate	Testoviron, Virormone	25-50 mg every 2-3 days (rarely available in USA)	Every 2-3 days	Europe, USA (rare)
Testosterone Undecanoate	Aveed (USA), Nebido (Europe, Canada, Australia)	1000 mg every 10 weeks	Every 10 weeks	USA, Canada, Europe, Australia

*Short acting options, such as testosterone propionate, are not readily available in most countries. On the other hand, long-acting options, such as testosterone undecanoate, can lead to long term fluctuations in testosterone levels.

For healthcare professionals:

Administration: It is important to administer an injection correctly to minimize any long-term risk of infection. The skin area should be cleaned properly with alcohol and repeat use vials should be cleaned with alcohol both before and after injection. The needle used to draw up the medication should not be the same as the needle used to inject. The vial should also be stored properly to ensure bacteria does not accumulate. Given that testosterone is carried in an oil-based compound (with the exception of testosterone suspension – which is not a TRT compound) it can be very slow to inject. A larger needle such as a 21g needle could be used to draw up the solution, and a 23g or 25g needle can be used for injection. Given that it is a multi-use vial, using a smaller needle is often preferable.

Doctors and other healthcare professionals should spend a couple sessions with patients reviewing proper injection techniques, including supervised injections, to ensure the patient has the appropriate skills before they self-administer at home.

Unexpected side effect: Localized inflammatory reactions can occur at the injection site. While sometimes these are infectious and can be cellulitis or a bacterial abscess, they are also often an inflammatory reaction to the compound itself. These are often self-limited and do not need any specific treatment. In some cases, corticosteroids can be used. A healthcare professional should always evaluate these and make the decision.

2. Patches

Description: Testosterone patches are applied to the skin and deliver a continuous, steady dose of testosterone. They are typically worn on the back, abdomen, or upper arm.

Benefits:
- **Ease of Use**: Patches are easy to apply and remove.
- **Steady Hormone Levels**: Patches provide a consistent release of testosterone, reducing fluctuations in hormone levels.

Considerations:
- **Skin Irritation**: Some individuals may experience skin irritation or allergic reactions at the patch site. This is a relatively common side effect that can be moderately severe.
- **Visibility**: Patches are visible and may be inconvenient for those who prefer discretion.
- **Dose Adjustments**: Patches are available in set doses, which can make it challenging to adjust your therapeutic dose.

Testosterone Patch Formulations

Formulation	Dosage	Dosage Range	Availability
Transdermal Patch (e.g., Androderm)	2 mg, 4 mg, or 6 mg patches applied once daily	2 to 6 mg/day (based on patch strength)	USA, Canada, Europe, Australia

3. Gels

Description: Testosterone gels are applied to the skin daily, usually on the shoulders, arms, or abdomen. The hormone is absorbed through the skin and into the bloodstream. It has a short half-life – as short as a couple of hours. This means that serum testosterone levels can decline very rapidly, which can be observed when blood tests are completed a few days after a dose. This often leads to confusion among doctors and patients when the testosterone level is low, despite recent use of testosterone topical gel.

Benefits:
- **Convenience**: Gels are easy to apply and integrate into daily routines.

Considerations:
- **Skin Contact**: Care must be taken to avoid transferring the gel to others through skin contact. Over time, this can pose a risk to everyone else in the household including children and pets.
- **Daily Application**: Gels require daily application, which may be cumbersome for some individuals.
- **Dose adjustments:** Dose adjustments can be difficult, nuanced, and unreliable.

Topical Testosterone Formulations

Formulation	Dosage	Dosage Range	Availability
1% Gel (e.g., AndroGel)	50 mg applied once daily	50 to 100 mg/day	USA, Canada, Europe, Australia
1.62% Gel (e.g., AndroGel 1.62%)	40.5 mg applied once daily	20.25 to 81 mg/day	USA, Canada, Europe, Australia
2% Gel (e.g., Fortesta)	40 mg (4 pump actuations) applied once daily	10 to 70 mg/day	USA, Canada, Australia (not widely available)
Transdermal Solution	60 mg (2 pump actuations) applied once daily	30 to 120 mg/day	USA, Canada, Europe, Australia

4. Pellets

Description: Testosterone pellets are small implants inserted under the skin, usually in the buttocks or hip area. They release testosterone gradually over several months.

Benefits:
- **Long-Lasting**: Pellets provide a long-term solution with a single insertion lasting 3 to 6 months.
- **Stable Hormone Levels**: Pellets offer consistent hormone levels with minimal fluctuations.

Considerations:
- **Surgical Procedure**: Insertion requires a minor surgical procedure, which may involve some discomfort.
- **Removal**: If side effects occur or adjustments are needed, pellets must be surgically removed.

Testosterone Pellets/Implants

Formulation	Brand Name(s)	Dosage	Administration Frequency	Availability (Regions)
Testosterone Pellets (Implants)	Testopel (USA)	150–450 mg (usually 6–12 pellets)	Every 3–6 months	USA, Europe, Australia

5. *Oral*

Description: Testosterone through oral consumption, as the name suggests, are pills used for testosterone replacement therapy. Traditionally, oral androgens pass through the liver due to 17a alkylation and become liver toxic. However, testosterone undecanoate does not induce any liver toxicity, which is why it is now available on the market in the form of an oral tablet and why it is a unique product.

Benefits: Naturally, pills are the easiest type of medication to consume.

Considerations: Frequent dosing, high prices, absorption variability and lack of clinical response in some have been general criticisms of this agent. Like many classes of medicines, a pill can alter a lab number but may not truly help the patient clinically and symptomatically.

Oral Testosterone Formulations

Formulation	Brand Name(s)	Dosage	Administration Frequency	Availability (Regions)
Testosterone Undecanoate (Oral)	Jatenzo (USA), Andriol (Canada, Europe)	120–160 mg per day (can vary)	Daily (divided doses)	USA, Canada, Europe, Australia

6. Intranasal

Description: Intranasal testosterone was approved by the FDA in 2014 and offered a convenient option for TRT.

Benefits: Naturally, the easy administration compared to injecting is a major upside

Considerations:
- The short half-life can create fluctuating levels of serum testosterone.
- Intranasal administration does not always provide consistent reliable absorption.
- Nasal allergies or irritation can be a deterrent for its use.
- Intranasal testosterone must be administered 3 times per day; this can be inconvenient for some and could even lead to missed doses.
- This novel formulation has a higher cost than other forms of testosterone.

Intranasal Testosterone Formulations

Formulation	Brand Name(s)	Dosage	Administration Frequency	Availability (Regions)
Testosterone Nasal Gel	Natesto (USA, Canada)	5.5 mg per nostril (total 11 mg) 3x daily	3 times per day	USA, Canada

7. Other:

Bio-identical hormone products: Bio-identical hormone products are processed hormones derived from plant materials. As the name states, they are identical to the hormones found in our bodies. While companies market these bio-identical hormones as natural, there is no large-scale evidence that bio-identical compounds have superior efficacy than traditional compounds.

Doctor's opinion: Injections continue to be the most effective and reliable method of treatment.

Risks and Side Effects of TRT

While TRT can provide significant benefits, like any other medical treatment, it is not without risks and potential side effects. Understanding these risks is essential for making an informed decision about treatment. The risks are generally misunderstood and, as of 2024, the evidence is not conclusive on many issues. However, in recent years, scientific evidence has shown that many traditional risk factors were incorrect. An important part of informed decision-making is to look at the entire body of evidence, consider that there may be unknown pieces, and then proceed.

1. Cardiovascular Risks?

Potential Risks: TRT has been a major discussion topic when it comes to cardiovascular health. But does it truly elevate the risk of heart disease? It depends on which studies you look at. There is generally no conclusive consensus on this issue, as some studies have shown no increase in cardiovascular disease with TRT whereas others have shown an increase. For many patients with truly low testosterone, recent studies have not shown an elevated risk of heart disease. What we do know is that there may be a shift in secondary indicators of risk such as cholesterol or hypertension. Some literature has shown an increased risk of atrial fibrillation as well. Again, we do not have a conclusive and definitive answer on this topic; maintaining that honesty is important.

Management: Monitoring cholesterol levels, blood pressure and other metabolic risk factors is the best way to minimize risk. Carefully monitoring these risk factors also makes it possible to start early intervention, when appropriate. Optimizing every lifestyle factor ahead of time is also important. For example, a decrease in saturated fat intake and increased cardiovascular exercise can offset some of the negative effects that exogenous testosterone has on the lipid profile.

Doctor's opinion: Genetics play a major role in this context. Many patients can use TRT and not have any noticeable change in their lipid profile for example. Others may see a substantial change. These differences are very likely explained by genetic differences.

2. Prostate Health?

Potential Risks: Testosterone can stimulate the growth of prostate tissue. While TRT does not cause prostate cancer, it can worsen benign prostatic hyperplasia (BPH) in some individuals. Pre-existing prostate cancer can also grow with TRT, if not undergoing active cancer treatment. Most recent and up to date evidence has shown that TRT is no longer considered a risk factor for developing new prostate cancer.

Management: For men who are middle aged, PSA monitoring (both total and free PSA) will be useful to minimize any theoretical risks. It is important to note that prostate cancer screening is indicated in all men in this age group, especially when considering the newest up to date evidence.

3. Sleep Apnea

Potential Risks: TRT may exacerbate sleep apnea, a condition characterized by interrupted breathing during sleep. There are multiple mechanisms by which this may happen with exogenous testosterone use.

Management: Patients with a history of sleep apnea should start treatment for their sleep apnea before starting TRT. Uncontrolled sleep apnea is considered a contraindication to TRT.

4. Skin Reactions & Acne

Potential Risks: Some TRT methods, particularly patches and gels, can cause skin irritation, rashes, or allergic reactions. Acne is also a well-known side effect of exogenous testosterone use but only in those with a genetic predisposition. More on acne later in the book.

Management: Switching to a different form of TRT or using topical treatments for irritation can help manage skin-related side effects. Acne can be treated with topical and oral agents, again, more on this later.

5. Fertility Issues

Potential Risks: TRT (and all exogenous anabolic androgenic hormones) can reduce sperm production and lead to infertility. This is due to the suppression of activity in the testicles, which affects sperm production. Notably, infertility is often temporary as sperm production usually restarts after discontinuation of the exogenous hormones.

Management: Men who wish to preserve immediate fertility should discuss alternative treatments or options with their physician, such as using human chorionic gonadotropin (hCG) alongside TRT. However, not everyone is going to experience fertility concerns when using TRT.

6. Polycythemia

Potential Risks: Some patients will get an elevated hemoglobin and hematocrit on TRT – essentially, your blood gets thicker. When this happens, it can increase the risk of thrombosis (deep vein thrombosis/pulmonary embolism) and other complications such as stroke. The level of risk is usually proportional to the degree of hemoglobin and hematocrit elevation. More on this at the end of this chapter.

Management: Therapeutic phlebotomy is an option for polycythemia, depending on the severity. Some patients may also benefit from daily baby aspirin, but this should be decided with one's physician. Discontinuation or dose reduction are also other options that need to be considered in some cases.

7. Acid Reflux / GERD

Potential Risks: For unclear reasons, exogenous testosterone use can lead to acid reflux in some users. Various theories exist, such as increased lower esophageal sphincter relaxation, which leads to increased reflux. However, none of the theories have been proven yet.

Management: The options would be treatment with a proton pump inhibitor (PPI), an H2 receptor antagonist such as famotidine, use of an antacid, dietary changes, or discontinuation of testosterone.

8. Other risks and abnormalities

- A **decrease in ferritin levels** is often seen due to a decline in hepcidin, as a result of exogenous testosterone. This can be misleading for doctors as it often presents a clinical picture of iron deficiency but without anemia. At least in the short term, iron stores may also become overutilized. This is also why it is important to obtain a baseline ferritin level so a comparison can be made during subsequent blood tests. More on this at the end of this chapter.
- There is a theoretical risk of **thrombosis** (deep venous thrombosis/pulmonary embolism) and those with a history of this must discuss it with their doctor. There has been mixed literature on this.
- **Water retention** is a possible side effect when starting TRT. Shifts in aldosterone and urinary sodium excretion can occur which leads to water retention. The potential result of this is high blood pressure. This can often be mitigated by control of dietary sodium intake, but some users may require diuretics and/or blood pressure medications.
- **Secondary hypogonadism** – Whenever exogenous testosterone is administered, the body shuts down its own testosterone production. If the user discontinues TRT, then they may or may not regain natural testosterone production. This can depend on the prior duration of use, dosages, genetics, age, and sometimes luck. For example, complete natural recovery of testosterone production is less likely if there is a history of prolonged TRT use for many years. However, if TRT was prescribed appropriately, then there is often significant pre-existing hypogonadism and that means baseline testosterone production

was already low to begin with. This makes it even less likely that natural production will recover adequately. But there are many common exceptions to this, like secondary hypogonadism, where TRT can be used temporarily until the underlying condition is treated.

- **Fatty liver** can occur in some patients who initiate TRT, especially if supraphysiologic levels are reached. This is simply due to the fact that being in a persistently anabolic state can lead to modest fat accumulation in the liver.

Monitoring and Adjustments

Effective management of TRT requires regular monitoring and adjustments to ensure optimal results and minimize side effects. Key aspects of monitoring include:

- **Hormone Levels**: Regular blood tests are necessary to monitor testosterone levels and adjust dosages as needed. Total and free testosterone levels need to be monitored to ensure the desired level is being achieved. Free testosterone is a key measurement as it indicates bioavailable testosterone, whereas total testosterone includes testosterone bound to sex hormone binding globulin (SHBG) and albumin bound testosterone. Monitoring of estradiol levels and prolactin is also useful, in case certain symptoms arise. It is ideal to monitor endocrine labs starting at 2 months intervals during the early stages of TRT. Then, depending on the prior results, spacing out the endocrine labs to every 6 months is generally recommended.
- **Symptom Assessment**: Ongoing evaluation of symptoms helps assess the effectiveness of the treatment and identify any adverse effects. If you have mid-range levels but still suffer from the same symptoms, the replacement dose may be inadequate. If the levels have risen quite significantly but symptoms persist, it is time to look for other causes of the symptoms.
- **Cardiovascular Health**: Monitoring lipid levels helps to see if the TRT is negatively affecting the lipids. HDL levels often decline with exogenous testosterone use and LDL levels can

modestly climb. Although, this does not happen in all patients. It is recommended to have baseline levels before starting TRT.
- **Hematologic Assessment**: A CBC provides you with the hemoglobin and hematocrit. Not all patients will get polycythemia, but some will. Again, a baseline CBC should be done.
- **Prostate Health**: For middle aged and older men, PSA level monitoring is generally important. Checking total and free PSA before starting TRT, then checking at regular intervals can provide insight into the PSA velocity while on TRT.
- **Bone Density**: Periodic bone density tests may be recommended to monitor bone health given that hypogonadism can often lead to osteoporosis.
- **Renal Function**: Creatinine levels should not climb on testosterone. However, elevated muscle mass can raise creatinine, and therefore cystatin C levels should be measured before and after for those on TRT.
- **Liver Enzymes**: TRT could possibly elevate the risk of developing fatty liver disease, though this is mostly dependent on pre-existing risk factors and genetics. Measuring liver enzymes before starting and then periodically on TRT can be useful. High levels should prompt a liver ultrasound and persistently elevated levels should always initiate a comprehensive liver workup.
- **Insulin resistance:** While TRT itself does not cause insulin resistance and diabetes and may even deflate hemoglobin A1C levels due to the induced polycythemia; patients with low testosterone often have metabolic risk factors. Therefore, screening for diabetes and insulin resistance would be recommended. To explain this concept in more laymen's terms, TRT can cause an elevated red blood count in some people. This abrupt change can cause an artificial manipulation of the hemoglobin A1C levels, which is a long-term measure of blood sugar and how we check for type 2 diabetes. If artificially inaccurate A1C levels are suspected, doctors can use the

fructosamine test which relies on albumin and not hemoglobin in order to measure blood sugar.

A Closer Look at Polycythemia and Low Ferritin

TRT can raise your hemoglobin and red blood cells while lowering your ferritin. This can be confusing and surprising at first, and the low ferritin can often be anxiety provoking. Doctors can mistake it for gastrointestinal bleeding and go down the wrong road in addressing the issue. Testosterone administered externally boosts the production of erythropoietin (EPO), a hormone that stimulates the bone marrow to produce more red blood cells. Alongside this RBC production, erythroferrone is generated. Erythroferrone plays a role in suppressing hepcidin, a regulator of iron metabolism. When hepcidin levels drop, ferroportin, a protein that controls iron release from cells, allows iron stored as ferritin to exit the cells more freely. This iron then binds to transferrin and is utilized in hemoglobin formation. Reduced hepcidin also prevents the usual storage of iron as ferritin, ensuring more available iron is directed into hemoglobin production for the bloodstream.

Once polycythemia develops, treatment comes down to its severity as well as the context of the person's clinical risk factors. Very mild polycythemia may not need treatment, but severe polycythemia, for example with a hemoglobin over 20g/dl (200 g/L), must be addressed. This may include therapeutic phlebotomy (removing blood). When this is done, ferritin levels can become depleted further. Notably, prolonged and excess iron supplementation can spike the hemoglobin further and create an endless cycle. While there is a lack of scientific evidence to provide guidance in this specific area, theories and protocols have been drafted. Specifically: frequent low dose iron supplementation for short time intervals. The hope is that this method provides modest ferritin repletion, in layman's terms, while avoiding any adverse effects. In terms of what to do with more moderate polycythemia, such as those with a hemoglobin in the range of 18.5g/dl (185 g/L), treatment protocols remain controversial. In some cases, aspirin 81mg (baby aspirin) can be used to minimize long-term risks. The decision on what to do should be discussed with one's TRT prescriber.

Exploring Aromatization and Estrogen
When starting a TRT regimen, one critical consideration is the process of aromatization, particularly in males with higher body fat levels. Aromatization refers to the conversion of testosterone into estrogen by the enzyme aromatase (see reaction below), which is more prevalent in adipose (fat) tissue. Overweight men, who typically have higher body fat, may experience increased aromatization due to the greater presence of this enzyme. Testosterone introduced during TRT may more readily convert into estrogen, potentially leading to symptoms such as water retention, gynecomastia (breast tissue enlargement), and mood changes. It is important to note that a large increase in estrogen is not universally experienced, but many men may experience this, so being aware of it is important.

Testosterone (T) → Aromatase (enzyme) → Estrogen (E2)

Significantly elevated estrogen levels can diminish some of the positive effects of testosterone therapy by impacting mood, libido, and overall well-being. Moreover, an imbalance in estrogen can disrupt the hypothalamic-pituitary-gonadal (HPG) axis, thus reducing TRT's effectiveness in improving energy and sexual function. In some cases, managing estrogen involves using aromatase inhibitors (AIs), which limit the conversion of testosterone to estrogen, thus maintaining a healthier balance between the two hormones. This is often an area where some users try to rely on others' anecdotal experiences rather than making a personalized decision. Monitoring estradiol levels, using the sensitive estradiol lab test, is important to be able to achieve this.

Now, it is also very important not to over-suppress estrogen, as low levels can also negatively affect health, particularly in terms of bone density, cardiovascular health, cholesterol, mood and sexual health. While it may be lesser known, estrogen plays an important role in maintaining bone strength and regulating mood, so careful monitoring of both testosterone and estrogen levels through regular blood tests is important. Managing this balance is particularly significant in men with higher body fat levels, who are more prone to hormonal imbalances due to increased aromatase activity.

Use of AIs has been somewhat controversial within the TRT community. The lack of evidence-based data has made it difficult to provide medical guidance. On the other hand, the benefits of estrogen are well known whereas the downsides of estrogen deficiency or high estrogen are also well known. It is clear that there needs to be a middle ground balanced approach. A reasonable potential method for men who are at higher risk of developing high estrogen levels on TRT, is the use of low dose AIs as a closely monitored approach to prevent estradiol levels from climbing too high. The decision to start an AI should always be made on a case-by-case basis and generally most people on TRT will not need to be on one at any point in time.

It is also important to monitor estrogen levels using the newer generation sensitive estradiol test to ensure false positives do not occur.

Pregnenolone
Pregnenolone is a steroidal precursor hormone synthesized primarily in the adrenal glands, brain, and gonads from cholesterol. It serves as an upstream component in the steroidogenesis pathway, acting as the raw material for the production of several other hormones, including progesterone, cortisol, testosterone, and estrogen. Pregnenolone also has direct effects on the nervous system, where it functions as a neurosteroid, modulating neurotransmitter activity and influencing brain function, including mood, memory, and stress responses. Due to its central role in hormone synthesis and its neurological actions, pregnenolone has been marketed as a supplement with various theoretical benefits.

Reviewing the Evidence

The evidence supporting pregnenolone supplementation remains limited and inconsistent. Some small studies and anecdotal reports suggest that it may improve memory, reduce stress, and enhance mood, potentially due to its neurosteroid activity and its role in modulating GABA and NMDA receptor systems. For example, preliminary research has indicated potential benefits in mood stabilization for patients with bipolar disorder or depression, but these findings are far from conclusive. In the realm of anti-aging, pregnenolone is often promoted for its supposed ability to replenish declining hormone levels, although no robust clinical evidence supports this claim. Furthermore, its impact on cognitive function in healthy individuals or those with neurodegenerative diseases like Alzheimer's is still speculative and needs more research.

While pregnenolone is generally considered safe at low doses, its supplementation is not without theoretical risks. Since it acts as a precursor to multiple hormones, supplementing pregnenolone can unpredictably affect downstream hormone levels, potentially leading to imbalances. Additionally, the quality and dosing of over-the-counter pregnenolone products vary significantly, raising concerns about consistency and safety. At this point, mainstream medical guidelines do not recommend pregnenolone supplementation for any specific condition due to insufficient evidence.

Chapter 7: Clomid, SERMs, and HCG

Clomid and SERMs

Clomiphene citrate, commonly known as Clomid, is a selective estrogen receptor modulator (SERM) that has long been used to treat infertility in women. In recent years, its utility in men's health has grown, particularly in the context of testosterone replacement therapy (TRT). Clomid blocks estrogen receptors in the hypothalamus, which leads to an increase in luteinizing hormone (LH) and follicle-stimulating hormone (FSH). This increase stimulates the testes to produce more testosterone naturally. It has become an appealing option for men who wish to raise their testosterone levels while maintaining fertility, as traditional TRT can lead to suppression of the hypothalamic-pituitary-gonadal axis which reduces sperm production.

The efficacy of Clomid in men with hypogonadism is supported by several studies. Research has shown that daily or every-other-day doses of clomiphene can significantly elevate serum testosterone levels, often doubling or tripling baseline levels within a few weeks. A study published in the *Journal of Sexual Medicine* reported that men treated with Clomid experienced a notable increase in testosterone without the usual side effects seen with exogenous testosterone supplementation, such as testicular atrophy. Clomid also avoids the challenges associated with testosterone injections, patches, or gels, such as fluctuations in hormone levels and the inconvenience of regular administration.

However, Clomid is not without its side effects; because it acts as a SERM, it can increase estrogen levels in some men, leading to symptoms such as mood swings, irritability, and even gynecomastia, in susceptible individuals. Other reported side effects include vision changes, headaches, and hot flashes, which can make prolonged use uncomfortable for some patients. While these side effects are not universal, they are significant enough that patients must be monitored closely during therapy. Regular blood tests are essential to ensure that estrogen levels do not rise too high.

Emclomiphene is an isomer of clomiphene that has been developed to address some of the limitations seen with traditional Clomid. Clomiphene is a mixture of two isomers: enclomiphene and zuclomiphene. Enclomiphene is primarily responsible for the positive effects on testosterone production, while zuclomiphene can accumulate in the body and contribute to adverse effects, such as elevated estrogenic activity and mood disturbances. Emclomiphene is a purified version of the active isomer, which aims to increase testosterone more effectively while minimizing estrogen-related side effects. This selective targeting makes emclomiphene a potentially more favorable option for men seeking to enhance their natural testosterone levels without the drawbacks of zuclomiphene.

The role of emclomiphene in treating hypogonadism is promising in some contexts, especially for men who want to avoid testosterone therapy or have imminent fertility concerns. Studies comparing emclomiphene to placebo have demonstrated its ability to significantly increase testosterone levels while maintaining normal sperm counts. Unlike exogenous testosterone, which can lead to the shutdown of the hypothalamic-pituitary-gonadal axis, emclomiphene helps stimulate the body's natural production pathways, preserving fertility. This characteristic makes it particularly appealing for younger men or those who are planning to conceive in the near future.

While the data on emclomiphene is still emerging, initial studies have shown that it has a more favorable side effect profile compared to the traditional clomiphene citrate. By eliminating the negative influence of zuclomiphene, emclomiphene reduces the risk of estrogen-related side effects, making it a potentially safer long-term option. However, more extensive clinical trials are needed to fully establish its efficacy and safety. For now, both Clomid and emclomiphene represent viable alternatives to traditional TRT, providing a way to boost testosterone while maintaining natural hormone production and fertility, but patient selection and careful monitoring are crucial to minimize risks and optimize outcomes. However, one important point about these medications is that sometimes the testosterone levels do improve on blood tests but the hypogonadism symptoms do not necessarily get better. This is a classic example of a medication that alters a blood test but does not necessarily change the final outcome.

In addition to clomiphene, other SERMs are sometimes used by men undergoing TRT to mitigate the side effects associated with elevated estrogen levels. Tamoxifen is one of the most used SERMs in this context. Originally developed for the treatment of breast cancer, tamoxifen works by blocking estrogen receptors, particularly in breast tissue, which helps prevent the development of gynecomastia—a condition that can occur when men on TRT experience elevated estrogen levels due to the aromatization of testosterone. While tamoxifen is effective at reducing estrogen's impact, its use in men also carries risks. Side effects can include vision changes, gastrointestinal issues, and increased risk of thromboembolic events, which is why caution is advised when using it outside of medical supervision.

Raloxifene is another SERM that has found use among men on TRT, particularly for those concerned with bone health and estrogen-related side effects. Raloxifene, like tamoxifen, blocks estrogen receptors but has a preferential effect on bone tissue, which means it can potentially support bone density while also reducing the risk of gynecomastia. The evidence for raloxifene's effectiveness in men on TRT is limited, but it has been used off-label in bodybuilding and hormone optimization communities. Side effects associated with raloxifene include an increased risk of blood clots, hot flashes, and leg cramps. These side effects, along with limited clinical research in men, underscore the need for careful consideration before using raloxifene as an adjunct to TRT.

Another SERM that has been used, though less commonly, is toremifene. Toremifene is structurally like tamoxifen and is used for the prevention of estrogenic side effects in men on TRT, particularly gynecomastia. The appeal of toremifene lies in its relatively favorable side effect profile compared to tamoxifen, but it is still associated with risks such as hot flashes, nausea, and the potential for cardiovascular issues. The use of toremifene in a non-clinical setting also lacks robust evidence and, like other SERMs, it requires careful monitoring to ensure that the benefits outweigh the risks.

HCG

Human Chorionic Gonadotropin (hCG) is a hormone that has a unique role in TRT. It mimics luteinizing hormone (LH) which is typically produced by the pituitary gland. LH stimulates the Leydig cells in the testes to produce testosterone. When men are on TRT, the body's natural production of LH is suppressed, which can lead to testicular shrinkage, decreased sperm production, and infertility. By using hCG, men can maintain testicular function, which helps preserve fertility and prevent atrophy while on exogenous testosterone. This makes hCG a valuable adjunct in the management of hypogonadism for some people, especially for men who want to maintain the ability to conceive while actively using exogenous testosterone.

hCG is typically administered via subcutaneous injection, and dosing varies depending on individual needs. It is often used two to three times per week in conjunction with TRT to maintain normal intratesticular function. The evidence supporting hCG's use in men undergoing TRT is relatively strong. Studies have demonstrated that hCG effectively stimulates endogenous testosterone production and helps preserve spermatogenesis during testosterone administration. In one notable study, men treated with both testosterone and hCG maintained adequate intratesticular testosterone, which is crucial for sperm production. This dual approach allows men to experience the benefits of TRT while mitigating the risk of impaired fertility.

However, hCG is not without its drawbacks. It can increase the body's overall production of testosterone and, subsequently, estrogen through the aromatization process. Elevated estrogen levels can lead to side effects such as gynecomastia, mood swings, and water retention, which may require additional interventions like aromatase inhibitors. While hCG can help maintain natural testicular function, improper dosing or self-administration without medical supervision can result in hormonal imbalances that negate the intended benefits. It is also essential to note that while hCG is commonly used off-label in the context of TRT, it is not universally accepted or approved for this purpose, and its use requires careful management to avoid potential complications.

The evidence for hCG as an adjunct to TRT is supported by both clinical trials and anecdotal reports from patients. Several studies highlight its ability to maintain fertility and natural testosterone production even when exogenous testosterone is introduced. However, individual responses can vary, and not all men may experience the same level of benefit. Its use should be closely monitored by healthcare providers, who can adjust the dose as needed to achieve optimal results without elevating estrogen to problematic levels. For men considering TRT, the decision to include hCG should be made based on individual goals, such as preserving fertility, and after thoroughly weighing the potential benefits against the risks.

Side Effects of hCG:
- Elevated estrogen levels which can lead to gynecomastia, in some users only
- Increased water retention
- Mood swings or irritability
- Headaches
- Injection site pain or irritation
- Potential for exacerbated hormonal imbalances, if not properly dosed
- Risk of testicular pain in some individuals
- Possible cardiovascular risks if very high estrogen levels occur and are not managed appropriately

Chapter 8: Understanding Gynecomastia

Gynecomastia is the enlargement of breast tissue in males due to an imbalance between estrogen and androgen levels. It is important to distinguish the difference between gynecomastia and pseudogynecomastia. While similar in appearance, pseudogynecomastia is due to excess fat while gynecomastia is characterized by the proliferation of glandular tissue. Gynecomastia can occur in one or both breasts and is often associated with tenderness or sensitivity in the affected area. While it is not an acutely dangerous condition on its own, it can cause self-esteem related issues and other psychological impacts. Long-term, there may be marginal risks in developing breast cancer. However, breast cancer in males is quite rare.

Causes of Gynecomastia

Gynecomastia has a wide range of potential causes, which can be classified into physiological, pathological, and drug-induced categories. Physiological gynecomastia often occurs during life stages associated with hormonal fluctuations, such as neonatal development, puberty, or aging. Pathological causes include conditions that alter the balance of estrogen and testosterone, such as hypogonadism, hyperthyroidism, chronic liver or kidney disease, tumors (testicular, adrenal, or pituitary), or genetic disorders like Klinefelter syndrome. Drug-induced gynecomastia is common and can result from medications like anti-androgens (e.g., finasteride – though relatively uncommon, and often at the 5mg dosages), anabolic steroids (the most common external etiology), antipsychotics, or medications that increase prolactin levels. Recreational drugs like alcohol, marijuana, and opioids can also contribute to gynecomastia, but are not primary causes. It is for that reason that it is important to consider all potential causes when evaluating gynecomastia.

Diagnostic Workup

Diagnosing gynecomastia begins with a detailed medical history and physical examination to differentiate it from pseudogynecomastia while also ruling out malignancy. Key blood tests include hormone panels such as total testosterone, free testosterone, estradiol, luteinizing hormone (LH), and follicle-stimulating hormone (FSH) to assess androgen and estrogen balance. Additional tests like thyroid function (TSH, free T4), liver function tests, and prolactin levels can identify secondary causes. In certain cases, imaging such as breast ultrasound or testicular ultrasound may be warranted to evaluate underlying abnormalities alongside other blood tests including AFP, LDH and serum HCG. If malignancy is suspected, mammography or biopsy might be necessary. The biggest mistake with this condition is automatically proceeding with a plastic surgeon referral without any due diligence of ruling out underlying causes. While most cases will be purely cosmetic in nature, it is crucial to ensure there is no underlying pathology.

Gynecomastia and Testosterone Use

Gynecomastia is a well-recognized side effect of anabolic steroid use or testosterone use, particularly when exogenous testosterone leads to significantly increased aromatization – the conversion of testosterone into estrogen. This process is facilitated by the enzyme aromatase, which is more active in individuals with higher body fat levels. Elevated estrogen levels stimulate the proliferation of breast tissue, resulting in gynecomastia. The risk is further increased when exogenous testosterone and androgen use suppresses endogenous testosterone production, thus disrupting the normal hormonal balance.

Treatment Options

Treatment depends on the underlying cause and severity of gynecomastia. For mild cases, observation may suffice, as gynecomastia can resolve spontaneously, particularly in adolescents. In persistent cases, medical treatments like selective estrogen receptor modulators (SERMs) (e.g., tamoxifen or raloxifene) are somewhat effective in blocking estrogen receptors in breast tissue, reducing glandular proliferation. Evidence supports their use in reducing gynecomastia, particularly in early stages, but they do not eliminate glandular tissue completely. Although, the literature has been somewhat conflicting on this topic.

For healthcare professionals: It would be appropriate to prescribe a SERM for some patients with gynecomastia, in a shared decision-making model. This is after a comprehensive workup is completed including thorough blood work and ultrasound, and for patients who absolutely want treatment but do not want a cosmetic surgery referral.

Aromatase inhibitors (e.g., anastrozole or letrozole) prevent the conversion of testosterone into estrogen and are useful in specific cases, though their efficacy is generally less robust than SERMs. Surgery, typically subcutaneous mastectomy, is the definitive treatment for severe gynecomastia. This approach provides excellent cosmetic outcomes and resolves symptoms permanently. Each treatment option must be carefully tailored to the individual, balancing effectiveness with potential side effects. Patient preference is also very important to highlight when selecting a treatment option.

Chapter 9: Acne – A Common Side Effect: A Review of Treatment Methods

Acne is a common skin condition that occurs when hair follicles become clogged with oil (sebum) and dead skin cells. It often manifests as pimples, blackheads, whiteheads, cysts, or nodules on the face, chest, back, and shoulders. Hormonal changes can be a trigger for the development of acne; as TRT results in hormonal changes, it can be a common cause of acne. Like many other conditions, some people are genetically predisposed to developing acne. That is why some may use testosterone and not develop acne, whereas others can develop very severe acne. One simple trick to identify whether acne development is a risk factor, is if the user had acne during the time period in which they went through puberty.

Given its significance as a major side effect of TRT and various PEDs, it is important to review what it is and how we can treat it.

Key Features of Acne:
Types of Lesions:

- Comedones: Open (blackheads) and closed (whiteheads) blocked pores.
- Papules: Small, red, tender bumps.
- Pustules: Pimples containing pus.
- Nodules: Large, solid, painful lumps beneath the skin.
- Cysts: Deep, painful, pus-filled lesions.

Causes:

- Excess oil production
- Clogged hair follicles by oil and dead skin cells.
- Bacteria: Propionibacterium acnes (now referred to as Cutibacterium acnes).
- Hormonal changes, particularly during puberty, menstruation, pregnancy, or stress.

Risk Factors:
- Genetics (family history of acne).
- Hormonal fluctuations.
- Diet (high glycemic index foods and dairy may exacerbate acne in some individuals).
- Certain medications (e.g., steroids, lithium).

Severity:
- Mild: Few pimples or blackheads.
- Moderate: More widespread pimples and possibly inflamed lesions.
- Severe: Numerous nodules or cysts causing significant inflammation and potential scarring.

The approach to treatment depends on personal preference, causation, severity and other risk factors. Treatments can include monotherapy or combination therapy with topical agents and/or oral medications. Here is an overview of available treatment methods:

1. Over-the-Counter (OTC) Treatments
Designed for mild to moderate acne. These will typically contain one of the following topical ingredients:
- **Benzoyl Peroxide**: Kills bacteria and reduces inflammation. This is the most common agent used in topical acne treatments.
- **Salicylic Acid**: Exfoliates the skin and unclogs pores.
- **Alpha Hydroxy Acids (AHAs)**: Promotes exfoliation (e.g., glycolic acid, lactic acid).
- **Adapalene Gel (0.1%)**: A mild retinoid for preventing and treating comedones.

Doctor's side note: Avoid fixating on brand names when it comes to acne treatments and instead look at the active ingredients.

2. Prescription Topical Treatments
Stronger formulations for moderate to severe acne, or sometimes for mild acne.

- **Retinoids**: Topical retinoids treat acne by increasing the rate of skin cell turnover, helping prevent clogged pores. Retinoid based prescription topical treatments include:
    - Tretinoin (Retin-A)
    - Adapalene (Differin, 0.3% for prescription)
    - Tazarotene (Tazorac)
- **Antibiotics**: Topical antibiotics treat acne by killing the acne causing bacteria. Antibiotic based prescription topical treatments include:
    - Clindamycin
    - Erythromycin
- **Combination Treatments**: These treatments combine the effects of topical retinoids and antibiotics to treat acne. These include:
    - Benzoyl Peroxide + Clindamycin
    - Benzoyl Peroxide + Adapalene
    - Tretinoin + Clindamycin
- **Azelaic Acid**: Reduces inflammation, kills bacteria, and helps with post-inflammatory hyperpigmentation.

3. Oral Medications

Recommended for moderate to severe acne or resistant cases. The options include:

- **Antibiotics**:
    - Doxycycline
    - Minocycline
- **Isotretinoin (previously known as "Accutane")**:
    - A powerful retinoid for severe, cystic, or treatment-resistant acne.
    - Requires close monitoring due to potentially severe side effects such as liver toxicity

There are numerous other treatment modalities such as chemical peels and laser therapy, but the intended focus is for common treatment options. TRT users can use a combination of topical and oral therapies depending on the severity of their acne and personal preference. The decisions regarding the optimal treatment plan should be made between the user and their doctor.

Isotretinoin – What's the big deal?

Isotretinoin, commonly recognized by most people by its former brand name Accutane, is a potent oral retinoid derived from vitamin A, primarily prescribed for severe, nodular acne that has not responded to other treatments. Introduced in the early 1980s, it truly was a "game changer" when it came to acne treatment by targeting the condition at its root cause. Unlike other therapies that aim to suppress symptoms, isotretinoin fundamentally reduces sebum production by shrinking sebaceous glands, limits bacterial proliferation, and modulates keratinization to prevent clogged pores. This multipronged approach makes it one of the most effective acne treatments available, often leading to long-term or even permanent remission in many patients. Over the years, its remarkable effectiveness has made it very popular. But it remains under scrutiny due to its well-documented side effect profile.

In clinical practice, isotretinoin is administered in weight-based doses, typically over a 5-6 month course. Patients undergo regular monitoring during treatment, including blood tests to assess liver function and lipid levels, as well as careful observation for side effects like dryness, nose bleeds, joint pain, and potential mood changes. As a side note, due to its teratogenicity, isotretinoin requires strict pregnancy prevention protocols, such as enrollment in programs like iPLEDGE in the United States, which mandates contraception and routine pregnancy testing for individuals who can become pregnant. It truly is a risk versus reward treatment option.

Doctor's Opinion: Isotretinoin (aka "Accutane"), works incredibly well at treating acne. However, there needs to be extensive due diligence to monitor side effects and lab abnormalities. For those who workout and train at a high intensity, they need to be careful about chronically elevated liver enzymes and elevated creatine kinase (CK) levels. Simultaneous use of isotretinoin and oral anabolic steroids should never happen.

Chapter 10: Access to Testosterone Replacement Therapy and Lifestyle Monitoring

Lifestyle Considerations

In addition to TRT, adopting a healthy lifestyle can enhance the benefits of treatment and support overall well-being. The biggest mistake many users make is not changing their lifestyle after starting TRT. So, while low testosterone levels warrant initiation of testosterone therapy, users often start TRT then present to their physician months later complaining of the same or similar symptoms. The reason? A lack of change in their lifestyle.

Key lifestyle considerations include:
- **Diet:** A balanced diet is the key to success. While certain diets may work for some, there is no "one size fits all" diet. A balanced diet that is ideal for your personal goals is what you should strive for. For those looking to gain muscle, consuming approximately 1 gram of protein per pound of bodyweight is ideal (for example: an individual that weighs 175 pounds consuming 175 grams of protein per day). This is alongside an intake of healthy fats and balanced carbohydrates while minimizing ultra-processed foods. More on diet later in the book, but the take home message is that transitioning from a packaged and processed diet to a balanced diet is the first key to success.
- **Exercise:** Regular physical activity, including weight lifting and cardiovascular exercise, is another staple requirement to enhance your results. Going from low testosterone levels to normal levels will set you up for success in the gym; this is something to take advantage of.
- **Sleep:** Adequate and quality sleep is crucial for hormonal balance and overall health. Establishing a regular sleep routine and addressing sleep issues can enhance the effectiveness of TRT. This includes addressing sleep apnea but also maintaining good sleep habits in general.
- **Stress Management:** Managing stress through relaxation techniques, mindfulness, or therapy can support mental health

and improve the overall effectiveness of TRT. This is especially true for those who have experienced poor mental health due to the adverse effects of low testosterone.

Patient and Healthcare Provider Collaboration

Successful TRT requires a collaborative approach between the patient and healthcare provider. Open communication and regular follow-up appointments are essential for:

- **Setting Realistic Goals**: Discussing treatment goals and expectations helps align the therapy with the patient's needs and preferences. TRT will not resolve every problem; in fact, it may not even be successful in addressing the patient's symptoms, especially nonspecific symptoms such as fatigue. It is also important to remember that not everyone responds equally; some patients see tremendous benefit after starting testosterone therapy while others see minimal benefit.
- **Addressing Concerns**: Addressing any concerns or side effects promptly ensures that adjustments can be made to optimize treatment outcomes. Remembering that scientific evidence is not perfect is key, as we do not know every single risk or risk level associated with TRT.

Barriers to Care and Online Clinics

TRT is increasingly recognized as a treatment option for men experiencing symptoms of low testosterone, yet it's still not universally embraced within medical communities. Only some doctors prescribe TRT or even feel comfortable following the care of patients who were prescribed TRT by a different doctor; this holds true in family medicine and various specialties such as endocrinology or urology. Many primary care physicians either lack specific training in hormone therapy or are hesitant to prescribe testosterone. This can be due to various reasons such as certain stigmas, outdated knowledge on side effect potential, or lack of knowledge on its benefits. Although, many physicians are excellent at recognizing this condition and immediately starting therapy once it is deemed necessary or making appropriate referrals. The last part is important to mention, given that medicine is a very large profession and not everyone is comfortable managing all conditions. Hence, referrals exist for that reason.

However, there is no perfect regional balance, and some patients are left without appropriate intervention. Consequently, men seeking TRT often face barriers when trying to find a way to initiate or continue therapy.

This hesitancy has led many men to explore online-only wellness clinics, which have emerged as a convenient, albeit controversial, option. These clinics often operate without the rigid oversight found in traditional medical settings, which can be both a benefit and a risk. The main benefit of these clinics is that they are more likely to approve and prescribe TRT compared to primary care physicians. This is good only for those patients with clinical hypogonadism who require TRT. However, convenience comes at the cost of a transactional approach to healthcare; the emphasis is frequently placed on quick consultations and fast prescriptions rather than a comprehensive medical evaluation. Patients using these services should usually (but not always) expect minimal physical assessments and generalized recommendations rather than individualized care. Online wellness clinics may also fixate on getting testosterone levels to a "target range" without addressing the patient holistically, potentially missing underlying health issues that could be contributing to symptoms. A great example would be a patient with a prolactinoma or hemochromatosis who has low testosterone and only receives testosterone therapy rather than a comprehensive evaluation. Again, to reiterate the key point, not all clinics function equally and there are good and bad options everywhere.

Another major consideration when pursuing TRT in Canada is the variability in insurance coverage, which can be both a logistical and financial obstacle. Depending on the province, public health insurance may not cover TRT in many instances, classifying it as non-essential unless hypogonadism is confirmed through rigorous testing and meeting certain thresholds. This leaves patients in some provinces to either pay out-of-pocket or seek private insurance that may, or may not, cover part of the cost. Moreover, the eligibility criteria for insurance coverage are often strict, requiring multiple tests and documentation of symptoms over an extended period, making the process arduous for those who could benefit from treatment. Even when private insurance does cover TRT, coverage often only extends to specific forms, such as injectables, while other methods such as topical gels may require additional expenses.

The hurdles with conventional TRT access and insurance have led many men to consider black market options. The availability of testosterone and other performance-enhancing drugs without a prescription is widespread online, and users are often lured by the ease of access, low cost, and claims of potency. However, this route is fraught with dangers, from inconsistent quality and unknown ingredients to the complete lack of medical supervision. Black market testosterone can contain contaminants or incorrect dosages, leading to potential health risks, which is noted in the chapter on anabolic steroids. The appeal of self-treatment often overshadows the reality that hormone therapy, without regular blood work and proper dosing, can lead to long-term health complications that outweigh any short-term benefits.

Despite these challenges, the landscape of TRT is gradually shifting. Awareness of low testosterone as a treatable medical condition and the benefits of appropriate testosterone therapy has grown in recent years. TRT is becoming more mainstream, with an increasing number of healthcare providers acknowledging its role in treating symptoms like fatigue, decreased libido, and muscle loss. The aging male population is driving the demand for treatment. While not every man will experience a decline in testosterone or will require testosterone supplementation, hypogonadism should be recognized as a condition that requires evaluation and treatment.

Chapter 11: A Look at Guidelines: What do Medical Societies Around the World Think about TRT?

Endocrine Society: The Endocrine Society recommends TRT only for men diagnosed with hypogonadism, confirmed by both clinical symptoms and consistently low testosterone levels on repeated tests. Diagnosis involves assessing total and free testosterone, as well as luteinizing hormone (LH) and follicle-stimulating hormone (FSH) to determine the underlying cause. The Endocrine Society emphasizes using testosterone therapy to alleviate symptoms like low libido, but not for individuals planning fertility or those with contraindications such as prostate cancer or uncontrolled heart failure. Regular monitoring should include testosterone levels, hematocrit, bone density, and PSA.

American Urological Association (AUA): The AUA guidelines advocate treating testosterone deficiency based on clinical symptoms and confirmed low testosterone levels. The treatment goals include improving symptoms, such as low libido and fatigue, and optimizing the patient's overall health. The AUA advises against blanket treatment of all men over age 65, instead recommending an individualized approach based on symptoms and risks. Monitoring should be carried out at 3 to 6 months after starting TRT, and assessments should include hematocrit, PSA, and liver function tests to detect side effects.

European Association of Urology (EAU): The EAU guidelines recommend TRT for men with clear symptoms of hypogonadism and low serum testosterone levels. Treatment decisions are based on the severity of symptoms and the patient's overall health, with particular caution in elderly men and those with cardiovascular risks. The guidelines recommend TRT for symptomatic relief but stress that testosterone levels should be measured in the morning, twice, to confirm the diagnosis. Monitoring includes regular assessment of hematocrit, lipid profile, PSA levels, and liver enzymes to mitigate potential complications.

International Society for Sexual Medicine (ISSM): The ISSM emphasizes that men with symptoms of testosterone deficiency and documented low levels should be considered for TRT. Treatment aims to improve sexual function, mood, and general quality of life. The ISSM stresses the importance of proper screening for hypogonadism, excluding other potential causes of symptoms. Monitoring should be conducted every 6-12 months, with specific focus on testosterone levels, sexual function, and screening for prostate issues, such as an increase in PSA levels.

British Society for Sexual Medicine (BSSM): The BSSM guidelines recommend using TRT for men with symptomatic testosterone deficiency after confirming low testosterone levels through morning testing. The goal is to alleviate symptoms such as fatigue, low mood, and sexual dysfunction. The BSSM guidelines advise regular blood tests for monitoring testosterone levels, hematocrit, PSA, and liver function. They emphasize the importance of a thorough patient history to rule out contraindications before starting TRT.

Canadian Urological Association (CUA): The CUA guidelines suggest diagnosing hypogonadism in men by evaluating clinical symptoms as well as two separate morning testosterone tests indicating low levels. The primary goal of treatment is to alleviate symptoms such as decreased libido and vitality. The CUA stresses that men with active prostate cancer or uncontrolled cardiovascular conditions should not receive TRT. Monitoring includes periodic assessments of testosterone levels, PSA, hematocrit, and overall symptom improvement, with adjustments made accordingly to ensure patient safety.

American College of Physicians (ACP): The ACP guidelines recommend TRT for men with low testosterone and symptoms that impact quality of life, such as sexual dysfunction. The guidelines advocate for shared decision-making, particularly discussing the risks, benefits, and long-term implications of therapy. TRT should be continued only if the patient reports significant improvement in symptoms, and treatment should be discontinued if no improvement is seen. Regular follow-ups, including testosterone levels and PSA, are recommended to ensure safety.

Australian Endocrine Society: The Australian Endocrine Society recommends TRT for men with confirmed testosterone deficiency and symptoms affecting their quality of life. Diagnosis involves both clinical assessment and repeated testosterone measurements. The guidelines stress that TRT is not recommended for men with uncontrolled heart disease or those who plan to father children soon. Ongoing monitoring involves regular assessments of testosterone levels, hematocrit, PSA, and cardiovascular health to evaluate therapy effectiveness and manage risks.

International Society for the Study of the Aging Male (ISSAM): ISSAM recommends TRT for symptomatic men with low testosterone levels, focusing on improving symptoms like sexual dysfunction, low mood, and muscle mass loss. The guidelines emphasize careful patient selection, particularly in older men, where the risk-benefit balance should be thoroughly discussed. ISSAM advises regular monitoring of testosterone, PSA, hematocrit, and cardiovascular health every 6-12 months, especially for elderly patients, to ensure safe continuation of therapy.

Asian Association of Andrology (AAA): The AAA provides guidelines on diagnosing and treating testosterone deficiency, emphasizing the importance of confirming the diagnosis with two morning testosterone measurements. Treatment aims to improve symptoms such as fatigue and decreased libido, with TRT considered only after discussing the risks and benefits. Monitoring recommendations include periodic evaluation of testosterone levels, hematocrit, PSA, and potential cardiovascular effects, ensuring the treatment remains safe and effective for the individual.

Germany - German Society of Endocrinology (Deutsche Gesellschaft für Endokrinologie): The German Society of Endocrinology recommends TRT for men with confirmed low testosterone levels and symptoms of hypogonadism. Diagnosis requires at least two morning measurements of testosterone, accompanied by clinical symptoms like decreased libido or fatigue. Treatment is considered on a case-by-case basis, particularly in older patients where risks must be carefully evaluated. Monitoring involves regular assessment of testosterone, hematocrit, PSA, and cardiovascular health markers. Men with active prostate cancer or severe cardiovascular disease are not considered candidates for TRT.

France - French Society of Andrology (Société Française d'Andrologie): The French Society of Andrology advises that TRT should only be used in men with clinical symptoms of testosterone deficiency and laboratory-confirmed low levels. Diagnosis involves assessing testosterone levels in the morning on two separate occasions. Treatment is recommended to alleviate symptoms such as low sexual desire and fatigue. Monitoring during TRT includes regularly checking hematocrit, PSA, and liver enzymes, with adjustments made as needed to ensure the treatment is both effective and safe. The guidelines also emphasize caution in men with cardiovascular conditions.

Italy - Italian Society of Endocrinology (Società Italiana di Endocrinologia): The Italian Society of Endocrinology's guidelines recommend that TRT should only be initiated in men with documented low testosterone levels and symptoms impacting quality of life. The diagnosis involves morning testosterone measurements and assessments of LH and FSH to determine the etiology of hypogonadism. Treatment is individualized, with a focus on improving symptoms like decreased libido and energy levels. Monitoring includes testosterone levels, hematocrit, lipid profile, PSA, and liver function tests to track treatment efficacy and identify any potential complications.

Spain - Spanish Society of Endocrinology and Nutrition (Sociedad Española de Endocrinología y Nutrición): The Spanish Society of Endocrinology and Nutrition recommends TRT for men with symptoms of testosterone deficiency and confirmed low levels on multiple morning tests. The guidelines emphasize shared decision-making between the physician and patient, especially for those with comorbidities like cardiovascular disease. Monitoring is conducted every six months and includes testosterone levels, PSA, and hematocrit to assess response to treatment and potential risks. The society advises against TRT in men who are actively trying to conceive or who have uncontrolled heart disease.

India - Indian Society for Bone and Mineral Research (ISBMR): The Indian Society for Bone and Mineral Research suggests TRT for men with low testosterone levels confirmed on at least two separate occasions and with clinical symptoms such as low energy and reduced sexual desire. The guidelines emphasize caution when considering TRT in men with high cardiovascular risk or prostate abnormalities. Monitoring involves regular testosterone level checks, hematocrit, lipid profile, and liver function tests. Additionally, the guidelines stress the importance of evaluating bone mineral density, as testosterone deficiency can contribute to bone loss and increased fracture risk.

Chapter 12: Erectile Dysfunction – When Testosterone is Not Enough

When experiencing erectile dysfunction (ED), low testosterone tends to be the primary suspected cause. Similarly, low libido tends to be blamed on low testosterone. However, as mentioned earlier, low testosterone is not always the culprit. While low testosterone can lead to ED, there are many other causes as well. In addition, restoring normal testosterone levels with TRT may not always solve ED. This chapter will list the various causes of erectile dysfunction as well as a variety of treatment methods.

Causes of Erectile Dysfunction
Erectile dysfunction can result from a variety of physical, psychological, and lifestyle factors. Below is a categorized list of potential causes:

1. Physical/Medical Causes
- **Cardiovascular Conditions**:
  o Atherosclerosis (narrowing of blood vessels)
  o Hypertension (high blood pressure) - as it can lead to vascular disease
  o High cholesterol - can be a cause of vascular disease
- **Endocrine Disorders**:
  o Diabetes (leads to nerve and blood vessel damage)
  o Low testosterone (hypogonadism) - Just one of many causes
  o Thyroid disorders (hyperthyroidism or hypothyroidism)
- **Neurological Disorders**:
  o Stroke - as it can co-exist with vascular disease but also cause significant neurologic deficits
  o Multiple sclerosis - can lead to neurologic deficits
  o Parkinson's disease
  o Spinal cord injuries

- **Urological Issues**:
  - Peyronie's disease (scar tissue causing curvature of the penis)
  - Prostate cancer treatments (surgery or radiation)
- **Chronic Diseases**:
  - Kidney disease
  - Liver disease - as it can alter endogenous hormones

2. Psychological Causes

- **Mental Health Conditions**:
  - Depression
  - Anxiety
  - Stress
  - Low self-esteem

3. Lifestyle Factors

- **Substance Use**:
  - Smoking (damages blood vessels and reduces blood flow)
  - Alcohol abuse (affects the nervous system and causes hormone balance issues)
  - Recreational drug use (e.g., cocaine, marijuana)
- **Diet and Exercise**:
  - Obesity (linked to reduced testosterone and blood flow issues)
  - Sedentary lifestyle (impairs vascular health)

4. Medications

- **Blood Pressure Medications**:
  - Beta-blockers
  - Diuretics
- **Antidepressants and Antipsychotics**:
  - Selective serotonin reuptake inhibitors (SSRIs)
  - Antipsychotics
- **Hormonal Treatments**:
  - Anti-androgens
  - Prostate cancer medications

- **Other Medications**:
    - Opioids (note that opioids can be a chronic cause of hypogonadism and ED)
    - Anti-seizure drugs

5. Hormonal Imbalances

- Low testosterone (hypogonadism)
- Excess prolactin (hyperprolactinemia)
- Elevated estrogen levels (e.g., due to obesity or liver issues)

6. Aging

- Natural decline in vascular health and hormone levels

7. Injury or Surgery

- Pelvic or spinal trauma
- Prostate surgery (radical prostatectomy)
- Bladder or rectal surgery

Treatment Options:

1. Oral Medications (PDE-5 Inhibitors)
Options:

- Sildenafil (Viagra)
- Tadalafil (Cialis)
- Vardenafil (Levitra, Staxyn)
- Avanafil (Stendra)

Availability & Access:

- Widely available by prescription.
- Generic options are cost-effective and accessible in most countries.
- Online telemedicine services often provide these medications after a virtual consultation.

Side Effects:

- Headache
- Flushing

- Nasal congestion
- Indigestion
- Back pain (tadalafil)
- Visual changes (sildenafil, vardenafil)
- Priapism (rare, prolonged erection requiring medical attention)

Doctor's Opinion: Viagra and Cialis are widely used for the treatment of ED and are 1st line interventions. Most common side effects are nasal congestion and mild headaches. While it may seem inconvenient and even embarrassing for some, these drugs are available by prescription only as some patients will have contraindications. These drugs are also recommended for those with psychologic causes of ED.

2. Lifestyle Modifications
Options:

- Regular exercise (improves cardiovascular health and testosterone levels)
- Weight loss for obesity
- Smoking cessation
- Reducing alcohol consumption
- Managing stress

Availability & Access: Freely accessible, requires personal commitment only

Side Effects: No direct side effects, but obviously requires consistent effort

3. Psychological Counseling or Sex Therapy
Options:

- Individual or couples counseling
- Therapy for performance anxiety, depression, or relationship issues

Availability & Access:

- Requires access to a qualified mental health professional or sex therapist.
- Increasing availability through online therapy platforms.

Side Effects: None, but success depends on patient participation and willingness.

4. Hormonal Therapy

Options: Testosterone Replacement Therapy (TRT) for hypogonadism (low testosterone)

Availability & Access:

- Requires a confirmed diagnosis of low testosterone otherwise TRT will not fix the ED
- More information on TRT can be found in previous chapters of this book

Side Effects: More information on TRT can be found in previous chapters of this book

5. Injectable Medications (Intracavernosal Therapy)
Options:

- Alprostadil (Caverject, Edex)
- Trimix (combination of alprostadil, phentolamine, and papaverine)

Availability & Access:

- Requires prescription and training for self-injection.
- Typically available at specialty pharmacies.

Side Effects:

- Penile pain or bruising
- Risk of priapism
- Scarring (fibrosis) with prolonged use

6. Urethral Suppositories

Options: Alprostadil urethral suppository (MUSE)

Availability & Access:

- Requires a prescription and is less commonly used.
- Can be expensive and less accessible than oral or injectable medications.

Side Effects:

- Urethral pain
- Mild bleeding
- Risk of priapism

7. Vacuum Erection Devices (VEDs)

Options: Mechanical pumps to create an erection by drawing blood into the penis

Availability & Access:

- Non-prescription devices are widely available online and in stores.
- High-quality, FDA-approved devices may require a prescription or professional recommendation.

Side Effects:

- Bruising
- Discomfort from constriction bands
- Numbness or cold sensation

8. Penile Implants (Surgical)

Options:

- Inflatable implants (three-piece devices)
- Malleable (semi-rigid) implants

Availability & Access:

- Requires surgical intervention by a urologist.

- Typically reserved for cases unresponsive to other treatments.
- Costly and often requires insurance approval.

Side Effects:

- Infection
- Mechanical failure (for inflatable devices)
- Loss of natural erectile function

9. Shockwave Therapy (Low-Intensity Extracorporeal Shock Wave Therapy - Li-ESWT)

Options: Non-invasive treatment using shockwaves to stimulate blood flow

Availability & Access:

- Offered at specialized clinics; not widely covered by insurance.
- Growing popularity but lacks universal accessibility.

Side Effects: Minimal: mild discomfort or bruising

10. Platelet-Rich Plasma (PRP) Therapy ("P-Shot")

Options: Injection of PRP into the penis to promote tissue regeneration

Availability & Access:

- Limited availability, offered primarily at specialized clinics.
- Considered experimental and not covered by insurance.
- Mixed data

Side Effects: Minimal: pain or swelling at the injection site

11. Stem Cell Therapy

Options: Experimental use of stem cells to regenerate penile tissue

Availability & Access:
- Limited to clinical trials or experimental clinics.
- Extremely expensive and not widely available.

Side Effects: Unknown, as long-term effects are still being studied.

12. Alternative Remedies

Options: Herbal supplements (e.g., ginseng, L-arginine, yohimbine)

Availability & Access:
- Readily available over-the-counter or online.
- Effectiveness is generally unproven, and quality may vary.

Side Effects: Vary depending on the product; some may interact with medications or cause allergic reactions.

13. Gene Therapy (Future Option)

Options: Experimental therapies targeting genetic factors affecting erectile function

Availability & Access: Currently only available in research settings or clinical trials.

Side Effects: Unknown, as research is ongoing.

Conclusion
ED is a condition with a wide range of causes, both physical and psychological. While hormonal causes, such as low testosterone, can contribute, many cases of ED are caused by cardiovascular disease, neurological illnesses, or lifestyle factors. Psychological components, including stress and anxiety, often exacerbate the condition.
Addressing ED requires a comprehensive approach that begins with identifying and treating underlying medical or psychological causes. Lifestyle modifications, such as improved diet, exercise, and stress management, can significantly improve outcomes. Medical treatments

from PDE-5 inhibitors to injectable medications and surgical options, offer effective solutions when lifestyle changes alone are insufficient.

Chapter 13: An Introduction to Anabolic Steroids and Performance Enhancing Drugs

Disclaimer: The following content on anabolic steroids, like any other content in this book, is strictly for educational purposes only and is intended to discourage anabolic steroid use. None of the information in the following chapters, or anywhere else in the book, should be used as medical advice of any kind in any context.

Introduction to Anabolic Steroids

Anabolic steroids are synthetic derivatives of testosterone and other agents, designed to enhance muscle growth, strength, and athletic performance. Though initially developed for medical use, anabolic steroids are often used in sports and bodybuilding for performance enhancement. This chapter will serve as an introduction to anabolic steroids and will be followed by chapters which will provide a comprehensive overview of major injectable and oral anabolic steroids, while highlighting the risks they present.

The use of anabolic steroids and performance-enhancing drugs (PEDs) has expanded significantly since their origin in Nazi Germany during the 1930s. It is speculated that German soldiers were administered these substances to boost aggression during combat. By the 1940s, Soviet and Eastern Bloc athletes began using them to enhance strength and performance. Over the following decades, steroid use became more widespread across various sports, leading to the International Olympic Committee officially banning anabolic steroids in 1976. This prohibition led to athletes seeking more creative ways to bypass detection, resulting in high-profile scandals like Ben Johnson's disqualification at the 1988 Olympics and the 2003 BALCO scandal, which implicated numerous well-known athletes. Today, anabolic steroids are illegal to possess in countries like the United States, though not illegal to possess in many other nations. Of course, they are prohibited in nearly all competitive sports.

Nowadays, both injectable and oral steroids are quite common for both recreational use and performance enhancement. Popular injectable steroids, like testosterone, are also used for TRT, except at much lower doses. Steroid users will use testosterone doses in the 500mg per week range, with some extreme users using doses significantly higher than that. Other commonly used steroids, such as the infamous trenbolone, are generally used in addition to testosterone. Trenbolone is considered a highly potent injectable steroid which poses some of the biggest health risks, such as kidney toxicity. On the other hand, oral steroids can cause liver toxicity and often can lead to extensive water retention. These compounds are traditionally cycled on and off, but some users will stay on certain exogenous compounds all year long.

How are they made and are they real?
Anabolic steroids are almost entirely manufactured on the black market. Raw powders are imported from foreign nations, and they are produced in the black market by various underground labs. The primary issues this can lead to is the variability in quality and safety. Many compounds can be underdosed or simply contain an entirely different compound altogether. This happens due to the ease of access to certain raw powders from overseas. A common example is the generic compound Oxandrolone, where it is sold under Anavar even though it is truly Winstrol or Dianabol. This can be very problematic for female users due to the vastly different androgenic properties of these compounds. Some compounds also contain high levels of heavy metals or other unsafe contaminants.

The Reality of Anabolic Steroids and PEDs: Deadly, Dangerous, or Safe?
The dramatic increase in deaths among younger bodybuilders as well as other individuals who were suspected of using PEDs has raised obvious concern about the risks of anabolic steroids. We know that anabolic steroids are inherently not safe to use and not directly beneficial for human physiology. We also know that they carry numerous risks. The real question is, just how dangerous are they? Like anything else, it depends.

The spike in sudden deaths has raised an alarm in the fitness community over the dangers of anabolic steroids. Anabolic agents, used at very high doses, can lead to coronary artery disease, heart failure, kidney and liver disease. Multi organ failure eventually sets in and, quite often, heart failure precipitates a lethal cardiac arrhythmia which then leads to sudden death. However, not all cases follow that pattern. Cardiac arrhythmias can also be induced by electrolyte abnormalities, which can occur following the improper use of diuretics – used by many bodybuilders for contest preparation. In addition, insulin misuse in bodybuilding can lead to a sudden and severe drop in blood sugar, which is acutely fatal if not treated emergently. Multi organ disease and heart failure can be exacerbated by various peptides and growth hormone used in the fitness community. Likewise, stimulants or thyroid hormone can also be precipitant for cardiac arrhythmia. In short, sudden deaths in the fitness community is a complex issue and is not solely isolated to anabolic androgenic steroid use.

There are also many factors such as genetics and preexisting risk factors that affect the health outcomes of users. This explains why there are many bodybuilders, who used various PEDs in the past, who are now much older without any known health concerns. On the other hand, there are many who unfortunately died young or suffer from severe organ disease at a relatively young age. While genetics are a key player in health outcomes following PED use, it is important to highlight that there is increased risk with greater abuse. Naturally, high doses of more dangerous compounds lead to higher risk. The most realistic point of view is to realize that it is ultimately a spectrum of risk that affects everyone differently.

Aging, Telomeres and Steroids
Telomeres, the protective caps at the ends of chromosomes, play a crucial role in cellular aging. Each time a cell divides, the telomeres shorten, and when they become very short, cells enter a state of programmed self-destruction. In summary, when the telomere gets too short, the cell dies. This progressive shortening is a key factor in the aging process and the development of age-related diseases.

Anabolic-androgenic steroids have been shown to further exacerbate telomere shortening. Recent research has also begun to explore the impact of anabolic steroids and exogenous testosterone on cellular aging, particularly concerning telomere length.

A study published in *Brain Sciences* investigated the effects of the anabolic steroid metandienone on telomere length in rats subjected to repetitive mild traumatic brain injury. The findings revealed that AAS administration led to a decrease in telomere length, suggesting that steroid use may accelerate cellular aging processes. Another study from *Molecular Ecology* published in 2021 showed that exogenous testosterone could accelerate telomere shortening. This research highlights the other potential long-term risks of anabolic steroid use, emphasizing the importance of understanding the broader implications of these substances on health and aging.

Chapter 14: Major Injectable Anabolic Steroids

Injectable anabolic steroids carry a much lower risk of liver toxicity compared to oral steroids. Below is a detailed look at various injectable steroids; some of which have or have had medical indications.

1. Testosterone Enanthate or Cypionate
Description: Testosterone enanthate is a long-acting form of testosterone with a half-life of approximately 4.5 days, whereas testosterone cypionate has a half-life of 8-9 days.

Common Dosage:
- **Medical Use**: 100 mg per week on average (can be up to 200mg weekly)
- **Performance Enhancement**: 250-750 mg per week (or more).

Cycles:
- Can last for 12 weeks, typically
- Some users do not stop using this agent and will instead "blast and cruise"; meaning that they will decrease their dose (cruise) following a period of high doses (blast), rather than discontinuing use between cycles.

Side Effects:
- Hair loss – for those with the predisposition only
- Polycythemia
- Dyslipidemia (low HDL is commonly seen)
- Acne
- Cardiovascular risks are associated with higher dose use of testosterone
- Thrombosis risks (though the risks are relatively low)
- Potential risk of atrial fibrillation

2. Testosterone Suspension
Description: Testosterone suspension is a fast-acting steroid with no medical use. It stays in the body for a few hours only; due to this, it

has been known to be utilized for doping with the purpose of evading drug tests.

Common Dosage:
- **Medical Use**: None
- **Performance Enhancement:** Commonly used doses are reported as being in the 50-100mg range. Frequency is multiple times per day or every other day.

Side Effects:
- Infection, given that suspension form is generally high risk for bacterial growth
- Aggression due to its abrupt and fast acting nature
- Similar potential side effects as with higher dose use of testosterone cypionate

3. Nandrolone Decanoate

Description: Known for staying in your body for longer periods, nandrolone decanoate has a long half-life of around 15 days. It was previously FDA approved in the United States for the treatment of anemia of chronic disease. It has medical use approval in various countries for the treatment of conditions such as anemia, wasting in HIV/AIDS, and osteoporosis. However, it is not a conventional treatment modality for any of these illnesses and does not have adequate research backing its safety. There are also reported benefits for joint pain.

Common Dosage:
- **Medical Use**: 50-100 mg once per week
- **Performance Enhancement:** 200-400 mg per week.

Side Effects (with higher doses):
- Decreased libido
- Erectile dysfunction – a common side effect
- Hair loss
- Increased risk of cardiovascular disease
- Mood changes

4. Trenbolone Acetate ("Tren")

Description: Trenbolone acetate is a powerful and infamous anabolic steroid known for its ability to promote rapid muscle mass and strength gains. It has strong anabolic and androgenic effects and numerous health risks. Trenbolone does not convert to estrogen, thereby reducing the risk of water retention and gynecomastia. However, it is known to be nephrotoxic, which means toxic to the kidneys. It is also among the most infamous anabolic steroids.

Medical Use: Trenbolone acetate is not approved for human use but has been used in veterinary settings to increase the muscle mass of cattle. It has never served any medical purpose in humans.

Side Effects:
- Aggression
- Night sweats
- Insomnia
- Kidney toxicity
- High blood pressure
- Suppression of natural testosterone
- Risk of cardiovascular disease
- Tachycardia
- Severe mood changes
- Focal segmental glomerulosclerosis (a rare kidney disease); can lead to advanced kidney failure, dialysis and the need for a kidney transplant

5. Boldenone Undecylenate (Equipoise)

Description: Boldenone undecylenate is a long-acting injectable steroid. It has moderate anabolic properties and low androgenic activity.

Medical Use: Boldenone has been primarily used in veterinary medicine to treat horses, improving appetite and physical condition. It has no medical indication in humans.

Side Effects:
- Increased appetite
- Water retention
- Possible anxiety
- Suppression of natural testosterone
- Elevated red blood cell count
- Kidney toxicity

Doctor's fun fact: Equipoise used to be a common steroid to test positive for in tested athletic competitions due to its long half-life and unreliable metabolism.

6. Trenbolone Enanthate
Description: Trenbolone enanthate is the longer-acting version of trenbolone, used for bulking and cutting cycles. It is highly anabolic and androgenic and has the same side effects as trenbolone acetate.

Medical Use: No approved medical use.

Side Effects:
- Aggression
- Insomnia
- Night sweats
- Cholesterol imbalance
- Increased cardiovascular risks
- Suppression of natural testosterone
- Kidney toxicity
- Focal segmental glomerulosclerosis / advanced kidney failure

7. Drostanolone Propionate (Masteron)
Description: Drostanolone propionate is a mild anabolic steroid primarily used during cutting cycles. It promotes muscle hardness and definition, often used by athletes and bodybuilders to achieve a lean, aesthetic physique.

Medical Use: Historically used to treat breast cancer in women, but not at present time.

Side Effects:
- Mild androgenic effects (acne, hair loss)
- Suppression of natural testosterone
- Cholesterol imbalance
- Low risk of water retention

8. Methenolone Enanthate (Primobolan)

Description: Methenolone enanthate is a mild anabolic steroid known for preserving muscle mass during cutting phases. It has low androgenic activity, with a lower risk of water retention and gynecomastia. To this day, it is commonly used inside the fitness community.

Medical Use: Historically studied for the treatment of breast cancer and anemia of chronic disease. It has no active medical use.

Dosages:
- Medical: 100–200 mg per week according to studied dosages, but again, not active medical indication.

Side Effects:
- Mild androgenic effects
- Suppression of natural testosterone
- Cholesterol imbalance
- Risk of hair loss (in those genetically predisposed)
- Polycythemia

9. Nandrolone Phenylpropionate (NPP)

Description: Nandrolone phenylpropionate is a faster-acting version of nandrolone decanoate. It has strong anabolic properties, mild androgenic activity, and has been reported to have positive effects for joint health (from a symptomatic standpoint).

Medical Use: Historically thought to benefit the treatment of anemia and muscle-wasting diseases.

Dosages:
- Medical: 25–100 mg per week.

Side Effects:
- Water retention
- Suppression of natural testosterone
- Gynecomastia
- Low libido
- Cholesterol imbalance
- Erectile dysfunction – one of the most common side effects
- Polycythemia

10. Boldenone Cypionate

Description: Boldenone cypionate is a long-acting injectable anabolic steroid, similar to Equipoise.

Medical Use: It has no medical indication for human use. Historically used in veterinary settings.

Side Effects:
- Increased appetite
- Water retention
- Possible anxiety
- Elevated red blood cell count
- Suppression of natural testosterone

11. Stenbolone Acetate

Description: Stenbolone acetate is an injectable anabolic steroid with moderate anabolic effects and low androgenic effects. It is used for lean muscle gains and cutting cycles without causing significant water retention.

Medical Use: Previously used to treat anemia and muscle-wasting diseases.

Side Effects:
- Suppression of natural testosterone
- Possible acne
- Cholesterol imbalance
- Polycythemia

12. Dromostanolone Enanthate

Description: Dromostanolone enanthate is the longer-acting version of Masteron. It is commonly used in cutting cycles to promote muscle hardness and improve muscle definition without causing significant water retention.

Medical Use: Previously used in breast cancer treatment.

Side Effects:
- Acne
- Hair loss
- Increased aggression
- Suppression of natural testosterone

13. Oxabolone

Description: Oxabolone is a less commonly known injectable anabolic steroid with both anabolic and androgenic properties. It is a derivative of nandrolone and was used in the past to aid in muscle growth and recovery.

Medical Use: No current approved medical use.

Side Effects:
- Water retention
- Suppression of natural testosterone
- Gynecomastia
- Cholesterol imbalance
- Acne

14. Oxymetholone - Injectable (aka Injectable Anadrol)

Description: Oxymetholone is usually taken orally but also has an injectable version. It is one of the most potent anabolic steroids in existence used for promoting rapid muscle mass and strength gains. It can lead to significant weight gain due to excess water retention. However, many users report feeling vaguely unwell while using it and suffering from fatigue and low appetite.

Medical Use: Used in the past to treat anemia and muscle-wasting conditions.

Side Effects:
- Severe liver toxicity (even in injectable form) though less toxic than the oral form
- Water retention – not as significantly as the oral form
- Gynecomastia
- Cholesterol imbalance
- Suppression of natural testosterone
- Low appetite
- Mood changes
- Polycythemia

15. Testosterone Decanoate

Description: Testosterone decanoate is a long-acting ester of testosterone, known for its slow-release properties. It is often used in testosterone blends such as Sustanon but can also be used individually for TRT.

Medical Use: Used for TRT for hypogonadal men.

Side Effects:
- Water retention
- Cholesterol imbalance
- Suppression of natural testosterone
- Acne
- Increased cardiovascular risks

16. Nandrolone Cypionate

Description: Nandrolone cypionate is a lesser-known esterified version of nandrolone. It has similar anabolic properties to nandrolone decanoate, but it is comprised of a different ester which affects its half-life and release time.

Medical Use: No approved medical use.

Side Effects:
- Suppression of natural testosterone
- Water retention
- Gynecomastia
- Low libido
- Cholesterol imbalance

17. Trenbolone Hexahydrobenzylcarbonate (Parabolan)

Description: Parabolan, also known as Trenbolone Hexahydrobenzylcarbonate, is a long-acting injectable form of trenbolone. It was developed for human use to treat muscle-wasting conditions but is now primarily used by athletes for its strong anabolic properties.

Medical Use: Originally developed for human use, but it no longer has approved medical applications.

Side Effects:
- Aggression
- Insomnia
- Night sweats
- Mood changes
- Increased cardiovascular risk
- Suppression of natural testosterone
- Kidney toxicity and advanced kidney failure

18. Methandriol Dipropionate (MAD or Methandriol Injectable)

Description: Methandriol dipropionate is an injectable anabolic steroid with both anabolic and androgenic properties. It has been used to enhance muscle growth and strength and is sometimes combined with other anabolic steroids to enhance effects.

Medical Use: Previously used for treating osteoporosis and wasting conditions.

Side Effects:
- Water retention
- Suppression of natural testosterone
- Liver stress (milder compared to oral forms)
- Cholesterol imbalance

19. Boldenone Acetate (Fast-acting Equipoise)
Description: Boldenone acetate is a shorter-acting version of Boldenone Undecylenate. It is often used in cutting cycles.

Medical Use: No approved medical use.

Side Effects:
- Increased appetite
- Cholesterol imbalance
- Suppression of natural testosterone
- Anxiety
- Mild water retention
- Polycythemia
- Possible kidney toxicity

20. Testosterone Phenylpropionate (TPP)
Description: Testosterone phenylpropionate is a medium-acting ester of testosterone, with a release time between that of propionate and cypionate. It was once a component of the Sustanon blend, but it can now be used on its own.

Medical Use: Used in the past for TRT.

Side Effects:
- Water retention

- Cholesterol imbalance
- Suppression of natural testosterone
- Acne
- Hair loss (in predisposed individuals)
- Polycythemia

21. Drostanolone Enanthate (Masteron Enanthate)

Description: Drostanolone enanthate is the longer-acting ester of Drostanolone (Masteron). It is primarily used in cutting cycles due to the lack of significant water retention.

Medical Use: Historically used to treat breast cancer in women.

Side Effects:
- Suppression of natural testosterone
- Cholesterol imbalance
- Acne
- Hair loss
- Polycythemia

22. Formebolone (Esiclene)

Description: Formebolone, also known by its brand name Esiclene, is an injectable anabolic steroid known for localized muscle swelling. Historically, it was used by bodybuilders shortly before a competition to enhance muscle definition.

Medical Use: No approved medical use.

Side Effects:
- Injection site pain and swelling
- Suppression of natural testosterone
- Cholesterol imbalance
- Mild water retention
- Polycythemia

Chapter 15: Major Oral Anabolic Steroids

Oral steroids differ from injectable steroids in many ways, such as potency and potential adverse effects. Notably, oral steroids generally carry an additional risk of liver toxicity. Below is a detailed look at various oral steroids:

1. Oxandrolone (Anavar)
Description: Oxandrolone is a milder oral anabolic steroid, popular for its low androgenic effects and popularity among female users. It is also known for having minimal water retention side effects. Oxandrolone is also less liver toxic than some other popular oral anabolic steroids. Since it is largely sold on the black market, it is sometimes faked, and another compound is substituted in its place.

Medical Use: Previously used to promote weight gain in patients recovering from severe burns, surgery, or chronic infections, and for osteoporosis treatment. It had FDA approval in the United States until 2022, which has since been withdrawn due to concerns of adverse effects.

Dosages:
- Medical: 2.5–20 mg per day.

Side Effects:
- Cholesterol imbalance, as it can cause a sharp decline in HDL levels
- Mild liver toxicity in some cases. An increase in liver enzymes is periodically seen.
- Suppression of natural testosterone
- Mild acne

2. Stanozolol (Winstrol)
Description: Stanozolol is a well-known oral and injectable anabolic steroid that has frequently been involved in doping cases.

Medical Use: Previously used to treat hereditary angioedema and promote muscle growth in patients with muscle-wasting diseases. It has FDA approval in the United States but is no longer marketed for any particular medical use.

Dosages:
- Medical: 2–6 mg per day (oral), 50 mg every 2–3 weeks (injectable).

Side Effects:
- Liver toxicity (oral only)
- Cholesterol imbalance
- Joint pains
- Suppression of natural testosterone
- Polycythemia
- Hypertension
- Left ventricular hypertrophy

3. Oxymetholone (Anadrol)

Description: Oxymetholone is a highly potent oral anabolic steroid, known for its ability to induce rapid muscle mass and strength gains as well as major water retention. It is often used in bulking cycles and is known for its high anabolic effects, though it also comes with significant side effects: it can be highly liver toxic, and users often complain of a general feeling of unwellness.

Medical Use: Used to treat anemia and muscle-wasting conditions.

Dosages:
- Medical: 50–150 mg per day were studied doses, but there are no active mainstream medical uses for oxymetholone

Side Effects:
- Severe liver toxicity
- Drug induced hepatitis
- Severe water retention
- Gynecomastia

- Suppression of natural testosterone
- Dyslipidemia – often severe
- Feeling unwell (a commonly reported side effect)
- Low appetite
- Polycythemia

4. Methandrostenolone (Dianabol)

Description: Methandrostenolone is one of the most popular and widely used oral anabolic steroids, known for its ability to rapidly increase muscle mass and strength. It is commonly used in bulking cycles but has significant estrogenic side effects. In some ways, it could be described as a milder version of oxymetholone, though it remains highly liver toxic.

Medical Use: Historically used to treat certain conditions of muscle wasting, but now has no active medical use indication.

Side Effects:
- Water retention
- Gynecomastia
- High blood pressure
- Liver toxicity, can be severe at high doses
- Cholesterol imbalance
- Suppression of natural testosterone
- Polycythemia

5. Methyltestosterone

Description: Methyltestosterone is an oral anabolic steroid used for TRT and performance enhancement. It is a synthetic derivative of testosterone and is known for its potent androgenic effects. It was widely available in the 2000s but has slowly become less common due to its liver toxicity effects becoming more well known.

Medical Use: Historically used in hormone replacement therapy for men with low testosterone and to help treat breast cancer in women. It is no longer used or recommended due to the liver toxicity.

Dosages:
- Medical: 10–50 mg per day were formerly studied doses.

Side Effects:
- Liver toxicity
- Acne
- Suppression of natural testosterone
- Water retention
- Dyslipidemia
- Polycythemia

6. Fluoxymesterone (Halotestin)

Description: Fluoxymesterone is a potent oral anabolic steroid with strong androgenic effects. It is used for strength gains and increased aggression but is not typically used for muscle mass gains due to its lack of anabolic effects. It has been considered a "dry" compound due to not inducing water retention.

Medical Use: Used in the past to treat male hypogonadism and delayed puberty, and in certain cases of breast cancer.

Dosages:
- Medical: 2–10 mg per day were formerly used doses

Side Effects:
- Severe liver toxicity
- Cholesterol imbalance
- Severe aggression
- Mood changes
- Suppression of natural testosterone
- Acne
- Polycythemia – if prolonged use

7. Mesterolone (Proviron)

Description: Mesterolone is an oral anabolic steroid with mild androgenic effects. It is used to promote muscle hardness and improve libido. It does not convert to estrogen and induces less water retention.

Medical Use: Used in the past to treat male hypogonadism and infertility.

Dosages:
- Medical: 25–75 mg per day were formerly studies dosages

Side Effects:
- Mild liver toxicity
- Acne
- Suppression of natural testosterone
- Dyslipidemia

8. Turinabol (Chlorodehydromethyltestosterone)

Description: Turinabol is an oral anabolic steroid which shares some properties with Dianabol, but it is considered to be less androgenic activity and cause less water retention. Like almost all oral steroids, it is liver toxic.

Medical Use: No approved medical use.

Side Effects:
- Liver toxicity
- Cholesterol imbalance
- Suppression of natural testosterone
- Mild acne
- Polycythemia

9. Metribolone (Methyltrienolone)

Description: Metribolone is an extremely potent oral anabolic steroid, considered the most powerful steroid. It has an exceptionally high anabolic-to-androgenic ratio and is used for muscle mass and strength gains. It is not widely available, due to severe toxicity concerns. It has also led to positive doping cases in the late 2000s.

Medical Use: No approved medical use due to its extreme hepatotoxicity. It was previously studied for the treatment of certain cases of breast cancer.

Side Effects:
- Severe liver toxicity
- Fulminant liver failure and death
- Kidney toxicity and advanced kidney failure
- Suppression of natural testosterone
- Cholesterol imbalance
- Aggression
- Prostate enlargement
- Polycythemia

Doctor's comment: This is the most dangerous steroid in the world.

10. Mibolerone (Cheque Drops)

Description: Mibolerone is an extremely potent oral anabolic steroid used primarily to increase aggression and strength in athletes. It is commonly taken shortly before competition but is highly toxic.

Medical Use: Originally developed for veterinary use to suppress estrus in female dogs.

Side Effects:
- Severe liver toxicity
- Aggression
- High blood pressure
- Dyslipidemia
- Suppression of natural testosterone
- Polycythemia
- Mood changes and depression

11. Methandriol Dipropionate

Description: Methandriol dipropionate is an injectable and oral anabolic steroid with moderate anabolic and androgenic effects.

Medical Use: Previously used to treat osteoporosis and muscle-wasting conditions.

Side Effects:
- Water retention
- Liver toxicity
- Cholesterol imbalance
- Suppression of natural testosterone
- Polycythemia

12. Desoxymethyltestosterone (Madol)

Description: Desoxymethyltestosterone, also known as Madol, is an oral anabolic steroid that was initially synthesized for potential pharmaceutical use but later became popular in sports for its strong anabolic effects.

Medical Use: No approved medical use.

Side Effects:
- Liver toxicity
- Cholesterol imbalance
- Suppression of natural testosterone
- Aggression
- Acne
- Polycythemia

13. Mestanolone

Description: Mestanolone is a potent androgenic oral anabolic steroid derived from dihydrotestosterone (DHT). It is known for its strong androgenic effects and its ability to increase aggression.

Medical Use: Used in the past to treat male hypogonadism. It has no active medical indication.

Side Effects:
- Liver toxicity
- Increased aggression

- Suppression of natural testosterone
- Acne
- Cholesterol imbalance
- Hair loss
- Mood changes

14. Methyldrostanolone (Superdrol)

Description: Methyldrostanolone, often marketed as Superdrol, is an extremely potent oral anabolic steroid known for its strong anabolic properties without significant water retention. It gained popularity due to its effectiveness in promoting rapid muscle gains.

Medical Use: No approved medical use.

Side Effects:
- Severe liver toxicity
- Cholesterol imbalance
- Suppression of natural testosterone
- Hair loss
- Polycythemia
- Hypertension
- Water retention

15. Quinbolone

Description: Quinbolone is an anabolic steroid intended for oral administration which is derived from boldenone. It was developed as a non-toxic alternative to other anabolic steroids, but its anabolic effects are relatively weak.

Medical Use: No current approved medical use.

Side Effects:
- Mild suppression of natural testosterone
- Possible liver stress (ex. Temporary increase in liver enzymes)

- Acne
- Hair loss

16. Furazabol (Miotolan)

Description: Furazabol is an oral anabolic steroid similar to stanozolol (Winstrol) with a reputation for promoting lean muscle gains without significant water retention.

Medical Use: No active medical use. Interestingly, showed potential therapeutic efficacy for dyslipidemia which is contrary to virtually all other anabolic steroids.

Side Effects:
- Liver toxicity
- Suppression of natural testosterone
- Hair loss
- Acne
- Polycythemia

17. Bolasterone

Description: Bolasterone is an oral anabolic steroid similar in structure to testosterone, known for its strong anabolic effects. It was initially developed in the 1960s and gained some popularity for muscle mass gains. It is no longer widely available.

Medical Use: No current approved medical use.

Side Effects:
- Liver toxicity
- Suppression of natural testosterone
- Cholesterol imbalance
- Acne
- Polycythemia

Chapter 16: Prohormones

Prohormones are a class of performance-enhancing drugs (PEDs) that serve as precursors to anabolic hormones, such as testosterone. They are designed to undergo enzymatic conversion in the body, which creates an active anabolic compound. Unlike traditional anabolic steroids, prohormones are inactive in their original form and only become active upon conversion. Historically, they were marketed as legal or safer alternatives to anabolic steroids. Prohormones were popular among athletes and bodybuilders for their ability to deliver performance benefits without the need for injections. However, their use is obviously not without risk, as they can cause significant side effects, including liver toxicity, hormonal imbalances, and suppression of natural testosterone production. In short, a similar story to anabolic steroids. Below is a detailed look at various prohormones:

1. Androstenedione

Description: Androstenedione is a prohormone that converts into testosterone in the body. It was a popular testosterone boosting supplement in the 1990s but was later banned due to health risks.

Medical Use: No current medical use. Previously marketed as a supplement for performance enhancement.

Side Effects:
- Suppression of natural testosterone
- Cholesterol imbalance
- Acne
- Hair loss

2. *1-Testosterone (Dihydroboldenone)*

Description: 1-Testosterone is a powerful prohormone known for its strong anabolic properties and mild androgenic effects. It is used to promote lean muscle mass and strength.

Medical Use: No approved medical use.

Side Effects:
- Suppression of natural testosterone
- Cholesterol imbalance
- Mild liver toxicity (oral form)
- Hair loss
- Acne
- Polycythemia

3. Dimethazine

Description: Dimethazine is a potent prohormone used in bulking cycles for muscle mass and strength gains. It is known for its strong anabolic effects but is also associated with liver toxicity. It has similar properties to superdrol.

Medical Use: No approved medical use.

Side Effects:
- Liver toxicity
- Suppression of natural testosterone
- Cholesterol imbalance
- Water retention
- Polycythemia
- Hypertension

4. Norbolethone

Description: Norbolethone is a synthetic prohormone originally developed for medical use which was later banned due to its adverse effects. It is known for its anabolic properties and was briefly used as a performance-enhancing drug.

Medical Use: Originally developed to treat malnutrition but withdrawn due to health risks.

Side Effects:
- Liver toxicity
- Cholesterol imbalance
- Suppression of natural testosterone
- Acne
- Polycythemia

5. 4-Androstenediol (4-AD)

Description: 4-Androstenediol is a prohormone that converts into testosterone after ingestion. It was popular due to its ability to increase muscle mass and strength but was later banned due to health concerns.

Medical Use: No current approved medical use.

Side Effects:
- Suppression of natural testosterone
- Cholesterol imbalance
- Acne
- Possible liver toxicity

6. 19-Norandrostenedione (Norandrostenedione)

Description: 19-Norandrostenedione is a prohormone that converts to nandrolone (19-nortestosterone). It is less androgenic than testosterone and was used for anabolic gains.

Medical Use: No current approved medical use.

Side Effects:
- Suppression of natural testosterone
- Potential mood changes
- Hair loss
- Gynecomastia

7. 1-Androsterone (1-DHEA)
Description: 1-Androsterone is a prohormone that converts to 1-testosterone in the body. It is used to promote lean muscle gains and is considered less estrogenic than other prohormones.

Medical Use: No approved medical use.

Side Effects:
- Suppression of natural testosterone
- Mild liver toxicity (oral form)
- Possible increase in blood pressure

8. Epistane
Description: Epistane is a derivative of dihydrotestosterone (DHT) known for its mild anabolic and anti-estrogenic properties. It has been used for gaining lean muscle mass and reducing estrogenic side effects. It does not lead to water retention.

Medical Use: No approved medical use.

Side Effects:
- Suppression of natural testosterone
- Liver toxicity
- Cholesterol imbalance
- Hair loss

9. Methoxygonadiene (Max LMG)
Description: Methoxygonadiene is an anabolic prohormone that is relatively non-methylated and used for muscle mass gains without significant liver toxicity. As with all oral compounds, the 17a methylation is what leads to liver toxicity.

Medical Use: No approved medical use.

Side Effects:
- Suppression of natural testosterone
- Potential for gynecomastia

- Cholesterol imbalance
- Bloating

10. 4-Androsterone (4-DHEA)
Description: 4-Androsterone is a prohormone that converts to testosterone in the body. It was used to help promote muscle mass and improve overall strength with fewer side effects compared to other compounds.

Medical Use: No approved medical use.

Side Effects:
- Suppression of natural testosterone
- Cholesterol imbalance
- Mild liver toxicity (oral form)
- Acne

11. M1,4ADD (Methyl-1,4-Androstenediol)
Description: M1,4ADD is a prohormone that converts to Dianabol (methandrostenolone), it is known for promoting rapid muscle mass and strength gains. It was commonly used during bulking phases.

Medical Use: No approved medical use.

Side Effects:
- Liver toxicity
- Suppression of natural testosterone
- Water retention
- Cholesterol imbalance
- Hypertension
- Polycythemia

12. Methylstenbolone
Description: Methylstenbolone is a powerful prohormone used to enhance muscle mass and strength. It was designed as an alternative to Superdrol, with similar effects but less liver toxicity.

Medical Use: No approved medical use.

Side Effects:
- Liver toxicity
- Suppression of natural testosterone
- Cholesterol imbalance
- Polycythemia
- Increased aggression

13. 13-Ethyl-3-Methoxy-Gona-2,5(10)-Diene-17-One (Max LMG)

Description: 13-Ethyl-3-Methoxy-Gona is a non-methylated prohormone used for lean muscle gains and mass building. It has a relatively milder effect on the liver when compared to methylated alternatives.

Medical Use: No approved medical use.

Side Effects:
- Suppression of natural testosterone
- Possible gynecomastia
- Cholesterol imbalance
- Bloating

14. Methyldiazolone (M-Drol)

Description: Methyldiazolone, often referred to as M-Drol, is a potent prohormone known for rapid muscle mass and strength increases. It is a variant of Superdrol, with high anabolic activity.

Medical Use: No approved medical use.

Side Effects:
- Significant liver toxicity
- Suppression of natural testosterone
- Cholesterol imbalance
- Acne and hair loss
- Polycythemia

Chapter 17: Steroids in the Clinical Setting: A Closer Look at Side Effects, Preventative Care, Medical Treatment and Common Lab Findings

Anabolic steroids have posed a significant challenge to healthcare providers for many years. Their development in the 20th century and widespread use in the 21st century have been linked to numerous health risks.

Assessing performance-enhancing substances can be challenging due to the wide variety of agents used. These range from anabolic steroids and peptide hormones to stimulants and beta blockers, among others. Usage patterns differ depending on the sport and the athlete's goals, but the most commonly used drugs are anabolic steroids and peptide hormones such as growth hormone. Anabolic steroids themselves can be categorized into testosterone-based steroids, classic synthetic compounds, veterinary steroids, and designer steroids. While many physicians are familiar with managing testosterone-based steroids, the use of synthetic and more exotic agents can fall outside their usual practice areas.

This underscores the need for physicians to be more vigilant and knowledgeable about these substances, enabling them to better manage and advise patients who may be using or considering performance-enhancing drugs. Physicians play a vital role in preventative care; addressing the needs of anabolic steroid users should be no exception.

What are the risks with anabolic androgenic steroids?
The use of anabolic steroids can lead to a broad range of side effects. These vary depending on the steroid type, dosage, and individual response.

For anabolic steroid users and patients: this is why being honest with your doctor can help guide what tests are done to ensure you are healthy and that a harm reduction strategy is being implemented.

For doctors: Familiarity with the specific steroids can help guide your medical decision making.

General Side Effects
- **Acne and skin issues**: Increased sebaceous gland activity leading to severe acne, oily skin, and cystic acne. Often only in those predisposed to it.
- **Water retention and bloating**: Steroids can cause the body to retain water, leading to puffiness and bloating. A lot of the rapid weight gain that is seen with steroids is due to water retention. This leads to rapid strength gains in a short period of time.
- **Gynecomastia**: Development of breast tissue in men due to the imbalance of hormones and increased estrogen levels because of aromatization. Usually occurs in those with a preexisting predisposition.
- **Mood swings**: Includes aggression, irritability, and "roid rage" (episodes of extreme anger or aggression). More prominent with certain steroids such as Trenbolone, and less so with just testosterone.
- **Psychiatric effects**: Anxiety, depression, mania, paranoia, or rarely hallucinations.
- **Suppressed natural testosterone**: Steroid use can suppress the body's natural testosterone production, leading to long-term hormonal imbalance.
- **Hair loss**: Increased risk of androgenic alopecia (male pattern baldness) in those with genetic predispositions. This occurs largely in DHT-based compounds and not all steroids.
- **Insomnia**: Difficulty falling asleep or staying asleep. Can be seen with all steroids.
- **Testicular atrophy**: Shrinkage of the testicles due to reduced testosterone production. This is usually a reversible side effect.
- **Libido changes**: Can cause increased or decreased sex drive. This will depend on the agent and the individual.
- **Increased risk of infections**: Due to the use of non-sterile needles or improper injections. This is a modifiable risk by the user.

- **Stretch marks**: Rapid muscle growth can lead to stretch marks on the skin.
- **Acid reflux:** Anabolic steroids can both induce and worsen acid reflux. Often it can be quite severe and refractory to therapy.
- **Worsened sleep apnea:** Various proposed mechanisms for why this happens.

Cardiovascular System

Steroid use can elevate the risk of cardiovascular problems. It is important to distinguish that there is no conclusive evidence that supports elevated cardiovascular disease risks in patients undergoing medically necessary TRT for hypogonadism. However, anabolic steroid use does carry numerous cardiac risks. Related risks include:

- **Hypertension (high blood pressure)**: This is generally seen with most anabolic steroids and is one of the most common side effects of steroid use. It is far more common with steroids that are known to lead to excessive water retention; hence oral steroids will be very likely to cause high blood pressure. However, it can happen with other compounds such as Trenbolone as well. This increases the risk of developing other cardiovascular concerns such as heart failure.
- **Cardiomyopathy**: Certain anabolic steroids can lead to left ventricular hypertrophy which can eventually lead to heart failure as well as sudden death. Coronary artery disease also can lead to heart failure in the long term. While cardiomyopathy can develop due to years of uncontrolled high blood pressure and coronary artery disease, it can also occur directly because of certain anabolic steroids. Winstrol or Stanozolol, as well as Trenbolone, can directly cause left ventricular hypertrophy.
- **Atherosclerosis**: Accelerated hardening of the arteries, which can increase the risk of heart attack and stroke.
- **Arrhythmias**: Irregular heartbeats, which can be dangerous depending on the rhythm. Atrial fibrillation risk does increase as a result of anabolic steroid use. Certain arrhythmias, such as

ventricular tachycardia (which can be imminently fatal), can occur as a result of severe left ventricular hypertrophy.
- **Increased cholesterol**: Elevated LDL ("bad" cholesterol) and Apolipoprotein B100 levels as well as decreased HDL ("good" cholesterol); thereby raising cardiovascular risk. The latter is most often seen, as exogenous anabolic hormones are widely known to cause suppression of HDL. Oral steroids are more likely than injectable steroids to cause a sharp decline of HDL.

Liver
Oral anabolic steroids, specifically, are known to affect the liver. It is considered the most common side effect of oral steroids specifically. This can include:
- **Hepatotoxicity**: An increase in liver enzymes, especially from oral anabolic steroids. The ALT, AST and GGT levels can all rise. GGT levels (traditionally thought to be associated with alcohol use) can have the sharpest increase amongst these 3 lab markers. Bilirubin levels can also rise in cases of clinically significant liver toxicity and drug induced hepatitis. This is most commonly seen with higher doses of Anadrol and Dianabol, among the more common steroids. Advanced cases could cause an elevation of INR, which can be a sign of liver failure. However, this remains uncommon.
- **Jaundice**: Yellowing of the skin and eyes due to liver dysfunction. This will correlate with bilirubin levels.
- **Hepatic tumors**: Development of liver tumors, which can be benign or malignant. Anadrol is most likely to cause this amongst the oral steroids.
- **Cholestasis**: Blockage of bile flow from the liver. A very high GGT level and bilirubin level will be seen, as well as high ALP levels.
- **Peliosis hepatis**: Blood-filled cysts in the liver.
- **Fatty liver disease:** This is the most common form of liver disease in Western nations, affecting up to 40% of the adult population in some US states. It is no surprise that it is the most common liver related side effect of any anabolic steroid as well

Any time there is a prolonged anabolic state in the body, there is the risk of fat accumulation in the liver.

Reproductive System

Anabolic steroids can significantly disrupt natural hormone levels. Once the body detects exogenous anabolic hormones, whether it be testosterone or another anabolic androgenic steroid, the hypothalamus will decrease the amount of Gonadotropin-releasing hormone (GnrH). This hormone generally tells the anterior pituitary gland to secrete Luteinizing hormone (LH) and Follicle stimulating hormone (FSH). These hormones communicate with the testes to produce testosterone. If there is less GnRH, then there is less LH/FSH and, therefore, less natural testosterone production.

In simple terms, anabolic steroids lead to the shutting down of natural testosterone production. However, testosterone and other steroids can undergo aromatization. This leads to the conversion of testosterone to estrogen. While these changes can seem like isolated numerical and biochemical changes, they can result in symptoms such as:

Men
- **Infertility**: Reduced sperm count and motility issues due to suppressed testosterone production, leading to difficulty conceiving.
- **Impotence**: Difficulty in maintaining an erection, prominent with steroids such as "Deca."
- **Prostate enlargement**: Can lead to urinary problems. This is most common among DHT based compounds.
- **Testicular Atrophy**: Shrinking of testicles due to decreased natural testosterone levels. This side effect is generally seen with any exogenous anabolic hormone.

Women

- **Virilization**: Development of male characteristics, including deepening of the voice, facial hair growth, and clitoral enlargement.
- **Menstrual irregularities**: Irregular or absent menstrual cycles.
- **Breast shrinkage**: Reduction in breast tissue due to hormone imbalance.
- **Infertility**: Disruption in ovulation and fertility.

Side note: While Oxandrolone, aka Anavar, remains one of the most common steroids used by women due to its low androgenic effects. It is often swapped with a different compound such as Winstrol or Dianabol. This leads to women unknowingly taking a highly androgenic compound.

Psychological Effects

- **Aggression ("Roid Rage")**: Increased irritability, hostility, or even violent behavior. Notably this is not a common side effect and does not occur with all steroids. Certain steroids such as Trenbolone or Halotestin are most likely to cause this. Testosterone can cause it at very high dosages as well.
- **Depression**: Risk of depressive symptoms or mood disorders, which will often occur when stopping steroids, particularly if there is a withdrawal of testosterone.
- **Mood changes:** Emotional instability and mood fluctuations. This includes episodes of elevated mood, hyperactivity, or euphoria.
- **Paranoia**: Irrational distrust or fear of others, but this remains a limited side effect. Most often this occurs with Trenbolone.
- **Addiction**: Psychological dependence on steroids, leading to compulsive use. However, steroids themselves do not cause primary addiction and do not cause legitimate cravings.

Endocrine System

- **Altered thyroid function**: Can suppress or stimulate thyroid activity, leading to thyroid dysfunction. This is often reversible and temporary.
- **Insulin resistance**: Can disrupt glucose metabolism, increasing the risk of diabetes. Insulin resistance remains an underappreciated risk with anabolic steroid use.
- **Hypercalcemia**: Increased calcium levels in the blood, but this is an uncommon side effect.

Musculoskeletal System

- **Premature epiphyseal plate closure**: In adolescents, anabolic steroids can prematurely close growth plates, stunting growth. This is one of the most important reasons for ensuring adolescents do not use PEDs. Simply put, starting anabolic steroids can immediately stop growth and prevent any height increase.
- **Tendon rupture**: Rapid muscle growth without corresponding tendon strength can increase the risk of tendon injuries. This is a major reason for some of the shockingly severe and unexpected injuries seen in Powerlifting.
- **Osteoporosis**: Long-term use can reduce bone density depending on the agent. Although, exogenous testosterone on its own does not cause this.
- **Muscle cramps**: Imbalance in electrolytes or rapid muscle growth can lead to cramping.
- **Joint Pain**: Some users experience joint pain or discomfort. This is most common among compounds that do not cause any water retention.

Immune System

- **Suppressed immune function**: Increased susceptibility to infections, usually viral ones. Most often occurs with testosterone specifically as users frequently report increased colds.

Kidneys

- **Kidney damage**: Long-term use can lead to kidney dysfunction or failure. Focal segmental glomerulosclerosis is a condition often cited which can occur due to trenbolone use specifically. Cases have also been reported while using Equipoise. It is important to check cystatin C levels and not solely rely on creatinine levels, which are often elevated in those with high levels of muscle mass despite normal kidney function.
- **Electrolyte imbalances**: Steroids can cause imbalances in sodium, potassium, and calcium depending on the agent. However, often these are minor alterations.

Other Side Effects

- **Fluid retention**: May lead to edema in some cases, also dependent on the specific agent
- **Increased body hair (hirsutism)**: Particularly in women but also in men
- **Changes in facial structure**: Overuse of steroids can alter facial features, making them appear more masculine in women or exaggerated in men. Especially prominent with trenbolone usage.
- **Impaired wound healing**: Slowed recovery from injuries.
- **Immune dysfunction**: Chronic use may suppress or dysregulate the immune system. More frequent viral upper respiratory infections (common colds) are noted in individuals who use anabolic steroids.
- **Low Ferritin levels:** Exogenous testosterone and many anabolic steroids suppress hepcidin which leads to laboratory evidence of iron depletion.
- **Headaches**: Persistent or severe headaches.
- **Polycythemia:** Elevated levels of hemoglobin and hematocrit which can lead to an increased risk of stroke and blood clots. This is one of the most common side effects of anabolic steroids.

Withdrawal Symptoms

- **Fatigue**: Tiredness when stopping use, generally due to the subsequent low natural testosterone levels
- **Depression**: Can be severe, particularly after long-term use.
- **Mood swings**: Irritability and emotional instability when discontinuing, variable from person to person
- **Loss of appetite**: Decreased interest in food.

What tests need to be performed for those using anabolic steroids?

This topic is very important for healthcare professionals. The answer to this question depends on the specific individual and which agents they are using. It is very important to distinguish anabolic steroid use from TRT and even the use of higher doses of testosterone. Considering whether an agent is injected versus consumed orally is important as they present categorically different risks, as mentioned earlier. Specific steroids can present unique health risks, so it is also important to consider the specific agents used. Dosages, usage of other performance enhancing drugs, and other agents like diuretics can also alter the management plan.

Every person who uses anabolic steroids should have a relatively comprehensive set of screening tests done, due to the broad range of risks involved. It is important to note that many anabolic steroids on the black market are not what they claim to be. Many times, they are a different agent which will still yield performance enhancing benefits. However, due to it being a different compound, this creates a challenge for practitioners looking to do screening tests. Hence, a broad set of screening tests remains the only realistic option.

A general panel of tests for all users would include:
- Complete blood count (CBC) to look for polycythemia
- Creatinine levels to assess kidney function
- Cystatin C levels to accurately assess kidney function. High levels of muscle mass artificially inflate creatinine levels, whereas Cystatin C is independent of muscle mass. This should always be ordered with creatinine levels. More on this later.

- Liver enzymes: AST, ALT, GGT, ALP – given the risk of hepatotoxicity with oral steroids, the risk of fatty liver disease risk with all steroids, and cholestatic liver disease risk, in some cases. It is a good idea to also check bilirubin, and reasonable to check INR levels as well.
- Electrolytes: sodium, potassium, calcium
- Ferritin levels: often on the low end of normal in all users due to hepcidin depletion. Low ferritin levels on their own, should not prompt a suspicion of gastrointestinal bleed unless there is another reason to suspect this.
- Hemoglobin A1C and fasting blood glucose: diabetes remains a risk as long-term steroid user can lead to the development of insulin resistance.
- Lipid panel to assess HDL and LDL levels.
- Apolipoprotein B100, which has been shown to be a critically important biomarker of lipid health. Also helpful if the triglycerides are high and the LDL cannot be accurately assessed.
- TSH and T4 screening given the potential effect of exogenous anabolic steroids on thyroid function
- Urine protein, through a urinalysis and urine protein : creatinine ratio, to assess for kidney disease. A complete urinalysis is also reasonable if the patient is using a compound that is known to be nephrotoxic.
- Electrocardiogram (ECG) screening is generally necessary given the inherent risk of heart disease associated with long-term anabolic steroid use

Going beyond general tests, there are numerous other tests that may be indicated depending on the user.

Lab tests:
- Lipoprotein (a): universal screening is recommended for everyone, but screening in patients already at a higher risk of heart disease is imperative as it would be an additional risk factor

- Total and free testosterone + LH/FSH levels: can be indicated if there is suspicion that the user is using entirely fake products, which is not that uncommon. LH and FSH would be the main markers to check as complete suppression is expected with exogenous hormone use.
- Fructosamine levels: obtained with an albumin level, can be very useful in confirming diabetes in patients with polycythemia given that the abnormal hemoglobin levels make hemoglobin A1C testing less reliable. This is especially true when there is a sudden spike in the hemoglobin levels after starting exogenous hormones. Fructosamine levels can then be converted to A1C levels using various available online charts. The main limiting factor is that frustosamine is a measure of the blood glucose in the past 3 weeks only.
- Total and free PSA levels: not usually necessary in patients under the age of 40 but it should be implemented into the testing protocol for patients above 40.
- Estradiol levels can sometimes climb quite high depending on the specific agent used
- Prolactin levels can also be elevated with anabolic steroid use and lead to numerous side effects, such as lactation.
- Fasting insulin and fasting blood glucose levels can be obtained to calculate a HOMA-IR level. While this is largely academic, it can expose developing insulin resistance and allow appropriate timely interventions to occur to prevent type 2 diabetes.

Cardiac testing:
- Echocardiogram testing is often indicated if the user has been on anabolic steroids for many years given the wide prevalence of associated cardiomyopathy. Any anabolic steroid user who has hypertension should strongly be considered for an echocardiogram. Long term chronic users should also have one done due to the risks of left ventricular hypertrophy.
- Stress tests can be indicated if the user has experienced any relevant symptoms such as exertional chest pain but also if the

physician has any general concern about the cardiac risks from long-term use.
- Coronary calcium screening would be an excellent test modality, especially if combined with a complete coronary CT scan, to exclude coronary artery disease. The main limiting factor for this test is the availability.

Imaging:
- Liver ultrasounds are commonly indicated as fatty liver disease is highly prevalent with anabolic steroid use. Both benign and malignant liver tumors can also occur with oral anabolic steroid use but are quite rare.
- Kidney ultrasound would be necessary if the user has an abnormal renal function on lab tests.

Doctor's side points: Fatty liver disease is quite common with anabolic steroid use. Excess exogenous anabolic hormones lead to greater glycogen storage and increased fat accumulation in the liver. Liver ultrasound and Fibroscan screening, pending liver enzyme evaluation, can be considered.

A Focus on Kidney Function and Muscle Mass: The story of abnormal creatinine levels

Perhaps the most common lab abnormality in those with a lot of muscle mass is high creatinine levels. The first assumption doctors make is to assume that the patient has kidney disease, when they see elevated creatinine levels. This leads to unnecessary workups, unnecessary referrals to nephrologists, and patient anxiety. It also leads to all sorts of factors being blamed such as creatine supplement use or steroids and PEDs that do not specifically harm the kidneys. This is all preventable with a slightly more nuanced approach to ordering lab tests on patients with a lot of muscle mass. This does not mean that high creatinine levels are always normal in these patients, it simply means that more information is needed.

What is serum creatinine?
Serum creatinine (the levels checked on blood tests) is a waste product produced by the muscles during the breakdown of creatine phosphate, a molecule involved in energy production. It is measured in the blood to assess kidney function, as healthy kidneys efficiently filter creatinine from the bloodstream into the urine. Elevated serum creatinine levels can indicate impaired kidney function or other conditions affecting renal filtration efficiency. So, the logical conclusion: higher serum creatinine levels must indicate kidney disease. Right? Not exactly and not always.

Why is serum creatinine elevated with higher muscle mass?
Serum creatinine levels are influenced by muscle mass since creatinine is a byproduct of creatine metabolism, which occurs in muscle tissue. Individuals with higher muscle mass produce more creatine and, consequently, more creatinine, leading to naturally higher baseline levels in their bloodstream. This physiological increase is not necessarily indicative of impaired kidney function but rather reflects the greater metabolic activity of larger muscle volumes. Therefore, when interpreting serum creatinine, it is important to consider factors such as muscle mass, alongside other markers. Without these other markers, it is not possible to interpret an elevated creatinine as normal or abnormal.

Which other markers are useful?
- Cystatin C - most important
- Urinalysis
- Urine protein:creatinine ratio
- 24 hour urine protein (if truly unsure)

What is Cystatin C and why is it so important in this context?
Cystatin C is a small protein produced by all nucleated cells in the body; it is released into the bloodstream at a constant rate. It is freely filtered by the glomeruli in the kidneys and almost entirely reabsorbed and metabolized by the renal tubules, making it a reliable marker for estimating kidney function. Unlike serum creatinine, cystatin C levels are not significantly influenced by muscle mass, diet, or gender,

making it a more precise measure of renal function in certain populations. It is particularly useful in detecting early stages of chronic kidney disease (CKD) when glomerular filtration rate (GFR) might not yet be significantly impaired. Measuring cystatin C can also enhance the accuracy of GFR estimates when used alongside creatinine-based calculations. This protein has become an important tool in nephrology for assessing renal function, especially in individuals with atypical creatinine levels or conditions affecting muscle mass, such as the elderly or those with elevated levels of muscle mass.

The main limiting variable for Cystatin C is that high body fat levels can affect its accuracy. That is why, for some patients, multiple tests are required.

Take home points for doctors:
Do not rely solely on creatinine levels to evaluate for kidney disease if the patient has a lot of muscle mass. This is true for those using steroids, not using any supplements at all, or those who take creatine among other supplements. Cystatin C should almost always be ordered during the first set of labs given the high prevalence of artificially elevated serum creatinine. If the results are inconsistent, then urinalysis and 24 urine protein analysis can be used to investigate further.

In the context of PED use, trenbolone is the primary compound that is known to directly cause kidney disease and extensive testing should be done for those who have used this compound.

Chapter 18: Drug use in Sports

The History of Doping in Sports

The history of drug use and doping in sports is as ancient as competitive athletics itself. Whenever a competition existed, there were also some methods developed to gain an edge over opponents. Early records from the ancient Greeks show that athletes used various natural stimulants to gain an edge in competitions. These enhancers were often plant-based extracts from herbs and fungi believed to enhance endurance, strength, and focus. Olympians in Greece, as early as 776 BC, reportedly consumed substances such as ground donkey hooves, opium, and even herbal concoctions to increase stamina. Roman gladiators followed a similar path, using stimulants and hallucinogens to reduce pain sensitivity and maintain high levels of aggression. These early forms of performance enhancements were widely accepted practices in ancient athletic circles, highlighting how long the pursuit of a competitive edge has existed in human history.

As athletic competitions evolved, so did the science of performance enhancement. In the 19th century, European athletes began experimenting with early synthetic stimulants, such as cocaine and strychnine, to gain energy and improve performance. By the late 1800s, cyclists, boxers, and endurance athletes frequently used these substances to fight fatigue and boost alertness during extended events. While these drugs offered short-term benefits, they also introduced new health risks, as athletes often experienced adverse effects ranging from nausea to fatal overdoses. Despite the dangers, no formal regulations existed, and athletes continued to use drugs largely unchecked.

The mid-20th century marked a turning point in doping with the development and introduction of anabolic steroids, which were synthesized in the 1930s to help treat conditions such as hypogonadism and delayed puberty. By the 1950s, Soviet Union and Eastern Bloc countries were rumored to use steroids systematically to boost athletic performance, particularly in strength-based sports such as weightlifting. This sparked a global "arms race" in sports, with Western countries quickly following suit. The Cold War era saw both sides heavily investing in doping research, aiming to demonstrate superiority not just in ideology but also in physical prowess. By the 1960s, anabolic steroids had become a staple in elite athletics worldwide, with athletes in track and field, weightlifting, and even professional football using these drugs extensively.

In response to mounting public concern over health risks and the integrity of competition, formal anti-doping measures began to emerge in the late 20th century. The International Olympic Committee (IOC) established the first official doping regulations in 1967, banning substances such as amphetamines and introducing testing protocols for anabolic steroids by 1976. Despite these efforts, enforcement proved challenging, as testing methods lagged behind the increasingly sophisticated ways athletes and coaches found to evade detection. High-profile scandals, such as the Ben Johnson doping case in the 1988 Olympics, brought doping to the forefront of public consciousness, forcing governing bodies to invest further in anti-doping technology and policy.

Entering the 21st century, doping has only become more complex with advances in pharmacology and biotechnology. The creation of the World Anti-Doping Agency (WADA) in 1999 marked a global effort to standardize anti-doping measures and close loopholes exploited in competitive sports. Despite these advancements, new doping methods including blood doping, synthetic hormones, and genetic enhancements, have emerged, challenging the limits of detection and regulation. Today, while sports organizations continue to battle the evolving landscape of performance enhancement, the allure of a competitive edge keeps doping an ever-present issue in sports.

It is worth noting that doping has become more challenging, as far as passing drug tests are concerned, due to the following factors: testing capabilities are more advanced than they used to, previously untestable drugs are now testable, and drug metabolism is not as predictable as some think, therefore metabolites may linger in the body for longer than expected.

Drug testing modalities

Drug testing modalities in sports have evolved significantly to keep pace with the sophistication of modern doping practices. Initially, testing was limited to simple urine tests aimed at detecting basic stimulants and anabolic steroids, but these methods quickly became inadequate as new drugs and masking agents were introduced. In response, governing bodies began refining and diversifying their approaches. Urine analysis remains a staple in anti-doping programs, but advancements now allow laboratories to detect not only the presence of drugs but also their metabolites, which can remain in the system longer than the drugs themselves. This level of detection has helped identify athletes using banned substances even after they have stopped taking them, increasing the chances of catching violations.

Another critical development in drug testing has been the adoption of blood testing, which allows for the detection of substances that may not be evident in urine alone. Blood testing is especially effective for identifying practices such as blood doping and the use of erythropoietin (EPO), which boosts red blood cell production to enhance endurance. Unlike urine tests, blood testing can measure changes in biological markers, providing insights into an athlete's natural physiological state and enabling detection of substances that might otherwise go unnoticed. This approach laid the groundwork for the "biological passport" system, which doesn't just test for substances at a single point in time but rather monitors athletes over an extended period, tracking variations in markers like hemoglobin levels. Abnormal shifts can indicate doping, even if specific drugs are not found in any individual test.

In recent years, anti-doping agencies have increasingly turned to new technologies like genetic testing and isotope-ratio mass spectrometry (IRMS) to detect and understand doping methods that exploit the cutting edge of biochemistry. IRMS, for example, helps differentiate synthetic from naturally produced hormones, which is crucial in identifying the misuse of testosterone and other anabolic steroids. Meanwhile, genetic testing has started to uncover cases of "gene doping," where athletes attempt to modify their DNA to enhance muscle growth, endurance, or recovery capacity. These innovations underscore a move toward precision and preventive monitoring, enabling sports authorities to address emerging doping threats proactively.

It is worth mentioning that blood tests yield very few positive results whereas urine tests continue to be the predominant testing modality to uncover doping. Blood testing is nuanced as many pathologies overlap with each other as well as with findings that are expected with doping cases. Urine testing makes it possible to evaluate general metabolites or even, with the use of advanced testing, the metabolites of targeted compounds.

Chapter 19: Performance Enhancing Drugs

Performance enhancing drugs (PEDs) are substances used to improve physical performance, endurance, or appearance beyond the typical limits of human ability. While anabolic steroids are often discussed, there are numerous other classes of PEDs that athletes and bodybuilders might use. This chapter explores selective androgen receptor modulators (SARMs), peptide hormones, insulin, diuretics, stimulants, erythropoietin (EPO), and insulin-like growth factor 1 (IGF-1), including their dosages, mechanisms of action, and potential side effects. While anabolic steroids also fall under the umbrella of PEDs, this chapter will not revisit them and will focus solely on the other categories of PEDs. The main reason for this is that the other types of PEDs fall under different categories in the context of medical care.

1. Selective Androgen Receptor Modulators (SARMs)

SARMs are a class of compounds designed to selectively target androgen receptors in order to produce muscle growth and fat loss. This selective mechanism is achieved through structural modifications that allow SARMs to modulate receptor activity uniquely in different tissues. While the downstream effects are similar to the effects of anabolic steroids, SARMs pose fewer potential side effects overall. For this reason, they are often marketed as safer alternatives to anabolic steroids. Though, their safety profile is questionable at best as they still pose numerous significant health risks. In addition, many compounds sold on the black market as SARMs are anabolic steroids fraudulently labeled as SARMs; this is very common in most countries.

Examples of SARMs

1.1 Ostarine (MK-2866)

Description: Ostarine is one of the most well-known SARMs, used for muscle preservation and growth. It has a half-life of approximately 24 hours, which has made it prevalent for doping in sports.

Side Effects:

- **Hormonal Imbalances**: Potential suppression of natural testosterone production.
- **Liver Toxicity**: Mild liver strain, though usually less severe than oral steroids.
- **Mood Changes**: Potential for mood swings and irritability.
- **Increased Cholesterol**: Possible negative impact on cholesterol levels.
- **Polycythemia**
- **Hypertension**

1.2 Ligandrol (LGD-4033)

Description: Ligandrol is another SARM used to increase muscle mass and strength. It has a half-life of approximately 24-36 hours.

Side Effects:
- **Hormonal Disruption**: May cause potent suppression of natural testosterone levels.
- **Liver Toxicity**: Mild liver strain with an increase in liver enzymes is quite common.
- **Gastrointestinal Issues**: Possible nausea or stomach discomfort.
- **Increased Risk of Hair Loss**: Potential to exacerbate androgenic alopecia.

1.3 Andarine (S4)

Description: Andarine is used for its muscle-building and fat-burning properties. It has a half-life of approximately 4-6 hours.

Side Effects:
- **Visual Disturbances**: Possible issues with vision, such as night blindness.
- **Hormonal Imbalance**: Potential suppression of testosterone production.
- **Liver Strain**: Mild risk of liver toxicity.
- **Increased Aggression**: Possible mood swings and increased aggression.

1.4 Cardarine (GW-501516)

Description: Cardarine is often used for endurance and fat loss rather than muscle gain. This is possible as it increases the body's ability to oxidize fatty acids.

Side Effects:
- **Liver Damage**: Long-term use may lead to liver toxicity, although this risk is still unknown
- **Potential for increased cancer risk**: Animal studies have suggested a potential link to cancer, warranting additional caution. This reason alone makes it important to avoid using this substance.

1.5 YK-11

Description: YK-11 is a SARM which is used for muscle growth and strength. It has a half-life of approximately 6-8 hours.

Side Effects:
- **Hormonal Imbalance**: Can suppress natural testosterone production.
- **Liver Toxicity**: Mild liver strain.
- **Mood Changes**: Possible changes in mood and aggression.
- **Hypertension**

1.6 RAD-140 (Testolone)

Description: RAD-140, also known as Testolone, is one of the most potent SARMs for increasing muscle mass and strength. It has a half-life of approximately 16-20 hours and is commonly used for bulking and strength cycles.

Side Effects:
- **Hormonal Imbalance:** Potential suppression of natural testosterone production.

- **Liver Toxicity:** Mild liver strain, though generally less severe than traditional anabolic steroids.
- **Increased Aggression:** Possible mood swings and irritability.
- **Headaches:** Reported by some users as a side effect.

1.7 S-23

Description: S-23 is a SARM known for its strong binding affinity to androgen receptors, leading to significant muscle mass increases. It has a half-life of approximately 12 hours and is also studied as a potential male contraceptive.

Side Effects:
- **Hormonal Imbalance:** High potential for suppression of natural testosterone production.
- **Testicular Atrophy:** Due to its contraceptive properties.
- **Liver Toxicity:** Mild liver stress may occur with use.
- **Mood Changes:** Increased aggression or irritability.

1.8 SR9011

Description: SR9011 is a compound often grouped with SARMs, but it is actually a Rev-ErbA agonist that affects circadian rhythm, metabolism, and endurance. It has a very short half-life of around 4 hours and is used for fat loss and increased stamina.

Side Effects:
- **Insomnia:** Due to its impact on circadian rhythm.
- **Increased Anxiety:** May cause restlessness or anxiety.
- **Hormonal Disruption:** Though not a direct SARM, it may impact hormone levels indirectly.
- **Mild Gastrointestinal Issues:** Possible nausea or stomach discomfort.

1.9 ACP-105

Description: ACP-105 is a newer SARM, often compared to Ostarine, with strong anabolic activity and a shorter half-life of around 4-6 hours. It is used to increase muscle mass and improve bone density.

Side Effects:
- **Hormonal Imbalance:** Can lead to suppression of natural testosterone levels.
- **Liver Toxicity:** Mild liver strain is possible.
- **Headaches:** Some users report headaches with use.
- **Increased Cholesterol:** Potential to negatively impact lipid profiles. It can cause sharp suppression of HDL (the good cholesterol).

1.10 LGD-3303

Description: LGD-3303 is a potent anabolic SARM that targets muscle and bone tissue, promoting muscle growth and improving bone density. It has a half-life of approximately 12-24 hours and is considered more anabolic than other SARMs like LGD-4033.

Side Effects:
- **Hormonal Suppression:** May suppress natural testosterone production.
- **Liver Toxicity:** Mild liver strain.
- **Increased Aggression:** Mood changes and irritability have been reported.
- **Cholesterol Imbalance:** May negatively affect lipid levels.

1.11 AC-262536

Description: AC-262536 is a relatively mild SARM with a lower affinity for androgen receptors. It is primarily used for muscle growth and fat loss, with fewer androgenic side effects.

Side Effects:
- **Hormonal Imbalance:** Potential suppression of natural testosterone.
- **Headaches:** Some users report headaches.

- **Liver Toxicity:** Mild, less frequent compared to more potent SARMs.
- **Mild Mood Changes:** Possible changes in mood or irritability.

1.12 BMS-564929

Description: BMS-564929 is a selective androgen receptor modulator that was developed with the purpose of increasing muscle mass and bone density in aging males. It has strong anabolic properties with minimal androgenic effects.

Side Effects:
- **Hormonal Imbalance:** Potential to suppress natural testosterone.
- **Liver Toxicity:** Mild liver strain may occur.
- **Increased Appetite:** Some users report increased hunger.
- **Sleep Disturbances:** Possible issues with sleep patterns.

1.13 JNJ-28330835

Description: JNJ-28330835 is an experimental SARM, studied for its ability to promote muscle growth and prevent muscle wasting. It has a strong anabolic effect on muscle tissue while being less androgenic.

Side Effects:
- **Hormonal Suppression:** Potential suppression of natural testosterone production.
- **Liver Toxicity:** Mild liver strain.
- **Mood Swings:** Potential for increased irritability or aggression.
- **Headaches:** Some users have reported experiencing headaches.

2. Peptide Hormones

Peptide hormones are short chains of amino acids that can stimulate various physiological processes. They are often used to promote muscle growth, fat loss, and recovery. Many have also been used for localized tissue healing or for presumed anti-aging effects. Generally, they do not directly induce the same anabolic properties that anabolic steroids do. Efficacy and side effect profile varies depending on the specific agent.

2.1 Human Growth Hormone (HGH)

Description: HGH, a very well-known peptide hormone, is used to stimulate growth, cell reproduction, and cell regeneration. It has a half-life of approximately 20-30 minutes in the bloodstream but effects last much longer. Historically, testing for HGH for doping proved to be challenging which made it prevalent for doping. Medically, HGH is used for certain conditions such as growth hormone deficiency.

Common Dosage:
- **Performance Enhancement**: The general dose used for performance enhancing purposes often starts at 2-4 IU (International Units) per day with much higher doses being commonly reported. Hence, more side effects can be seen as HGH often has a dose dependent response.
- **Medical Use**: 1-2 IU per day.

Side Effects:
- **Joint Pain:** Common side effect due to fluid retention.
- **Carpal Tunnel Syndrome:** Increased risk due to swelling of tissues.
- **Insulin Resistance:** Potential for development of type 2 diabetes. This is a common adverse effect.
- **Acromegaly:** Excessive growth of bones and tissues in adults.
- **Edema:** Fluid retention leading to swelling.
- **Cancer risk:** HGH can lead to the growth of all cells, including any preexisting cancer cells in the body. These are cells that may have been eradicated by the body, but now can grow further due to HGH.

2.2 Insulin

Description: Insulin is a hormone that regulates glucose levels in the blood. It is widely used in medicine for the treatment of insulin-dependent diabetes. In sports, it has been used to enhance nutrient uptake and recovery but is often abused for its anabolic effects. Insulin is generally considered one of the riskiest substances to utilize for performance enhancement due to the risk of hypoglycemia (low blood sugar) which can be fatal. A dose that is a little bit too high, or lack of immediate carbohydrate intake, can lead to death.

Side Effects:
- **Hypoglycemia:** Dangerous drop in blood sugar levels, which can cause dizziness, confusion, and loss of consciousness.
- **Weight Gain:** Increased fat accumulation if not managed with proper diet and exercise.
- **Insulin Resistance:** Long-term use can lead to decreased sensitivity to insulin and the development of type 2 diabetes. This is quite common amongst those who use insulin long-term for performance enhancement purposes.

2.3 IGF-1 (Insulin-like Growth Factor 1)
Description: IGF-1 is involved in growth and development, with effects similar to HGH but more localized. It is FDA approved for medical use in the United States, for those with growth failure.

Side Effects:
- **Joint Pain:** Similar to HGH, can cause discomfort in the joints.
- **Increased Risk of Cancer:** Potential to promote cancer cell growth.
- **Insulin Resistance:** Can exacerbate insulin resistance and increase risk of diabetes.
- **Fluid Retention:** Potential for edema.

2.4 GHRP-6 (Growth Hormone Releasing Peptide-6)
Description: GHRP-6 is a synthetic growth hormone-releasing peptide that is used to increase the body's natural production of growth hormone. It has a half-life of approximately 20-30 minutes and is often used in the fitness industry for muscle growth and recovery.

Side Effects:

- **Increased Hunger:** GHRP-6 is known for stimulating ghrelin, leading to increased appetite.
- **Water Retention:** Possible fluid retention may occur.
- **Lethargy:** Some users report feeling tired after administration.
- **Potential Insulin Resistance:** Long-term use could potentially impact insulin sensitivity and lead to type 2 diabetes.

2.5 GHRP-2 (Growth Hormone Releasing Peptide-2)

Description: GHRP-2 is another synthetic growth hormone-releasing peptide used for increasing natural growth hormone production. It is similar to GHRP-6 but has a stronger effect on GH release. It has a half-life of around 15-30 minutes.

Side Effects:
- **Increased Cortisol:** Can raise cortisol levels, leading to potential stress and anxiety.
- **Increased Prolactin:** Potential for elevated prolactin levels.
- **Hunger:** Similar to GHRP-6, it can increase hunger.
- **Water Retention:** Fluid retention may occur.

2.6 CJC-1295 (Modified GRF 1-29)

Description: CJC-1295 is a growth hormone-releasing hormone (GHRH) analog used to stimulate the pituitary gland to release more growth hormone. It has a longer half-life of approximately 6-8 days due to its ability to bind to albumin, which prolongs its activity.

Side Effects:
- **Injection Site Reactions:** Redness or swelling at the injection site.
- **Water Retention:** Some users may experience fluid retention.
- **Numbness or Tingling:** Possible tingling in the extremities.
- **Lethargy:** Fatigue may occur as a side effect.

2.7 Melanotan II

Description: Melanotan II is a synthetic analog of the melanocyte-stimulating hormone (MSH) and is used for promoting tanning of the skin. It is also used for increasing libido and erectile function.

Side Effects:
- **Nausea:** Common side effect, especially after the initial dose.
- **Darkened Moles:** May cause existing moles to darken.
- **Increased Libido:** Some users report heightened libido.
- **Injection Site Reactions:** Possible irritation or redness at the site of injection.

2.8 TB-500 (Thymosin Beta-4)
Description: TB-500 is a synthetic version of a naturally occurring peptide, thymosin beta-4, used to promote healing and recovery. It is used in the fitness industry for its potential to accelerate recovery from injuries. This compound should be studied further.

Side Effects:
- **Dizziness:** Some users report feeling lightheaded.
- **Injection Site Reactions:** Swelling or irritation may occur.
- **Lethargy:** Potential fatigue post-injection.
- **Immune System Effects:** Possible suppression of immune response with long-term use.

2.9 BPC-157 (Body Protection Compound)
Description: BPC-157 is a synthetic peptide derived from a protective protein found in the stomach. It is used for accelerating the healing of injuries, particularly in tendons and ligaments.

Side Effects:
- **Nausea:** Some users report feeling nauseous.
- **Injection Site Reactions:** Redness or discomfort at the site of injection.
- **Dizziness:** Mild dizziness may occur.

- **Possible Immune Suppression:** With extended use, there could be effects on the immune system.

2.10 Follistatin

Description: Follistatin is a naturally occurring protein that inhibits myostatin, a growth factor that limits muscle growth. It is used in the fitness industry for increasing muscle mass by reducing myostatin's inhibitory effect.

Side Effects:
- **Joint Pain:** Some users report joint discomfort.
- **Muscle Stiffness:** Increased muscle stiffness has been noted.
- **Injection Site Reactions:** Irritation or swelling at the injection site.
- **Hormonal Disruption:** Potential for unintended effects on hormone regulation.

2.11 Hexarelin

Description: Hexarelin is a synthetic growth hormone-releasing peptide similar to GHRP-6, used for promoting growth hormone secretion. It has a half-life of approximately 30 minutes and is used in the fitness industry for muscle growth and fat loss.

Side Effects:
- **Increased Prolactin Levels:** May cause elevated prolactin.
- **Water Retention:** Fluid retention is common with use.
- **Lethargy:** Fatigue or drowsiness may occur.
- **Heart Effects:** Potential for negative cardiovascular effects with long-term use.

2.12 Tesamorelin

Description: Tesamorelin is a synthetic analog of growth hormone-releasing hormone (GHRH) used for stimulating growth hormone production. It is also used in medical settings for reducing visceral fat in HIV patients.

Side Effects:

- **Injection Site Reactions:** Redness or irritation at the injection site.
- **Joint Pain:** Possible joint discomfort.
- **Water Retention:** Fluid retention may occur.
- **Increased Blood Sugar:** Potential effect on insulin sensitivity.

2.13 Selank

Description: Selank is a synthetic peptide developed for its anti-anxiety and nootropic effects. It is used for reducing anxiety and improving cognitive function.

Side Effects:
- **Drowsiness**: Some users report feeling sleepy after administration.
- **Dry Mouth:** Possible dryness of the mouth.
- **Injection Site Reactions:** Mild irritation or redness.
- **Headaches:** Some users may experience headaches.

2.14 MK-677 (Ibutamoren)

Description: MK-677, also known as Ibutamoren, is a growth hormone secretagogue used for increasing growth hormone and IGF-1 levels. It is popular in the fitness industry for muscle growth, fat loss, and recovery. Unlike other peptides, it is taken orally.

Side Effects:
- **Increased Appetite:** MK-677 is known for significantly stimulating hunger.
- **Water Retention:** Possible fluid retention.
- **Lethargy:** Fatigue may occur, especially during the first few weeks.
- **Increased Blood Sugar:** Potential for elevated blood sugar or reduced insulin sensitivity.

3. Diuretics

Diuretics are used to increase urine production and reduce fluid retention, often used by bodybuilders to achieve a "cut" appearance by eliminating water retention. However, diuretics can cause electrolyte abnormalities such as hypokalemia (low potassium) or hyponatremia (low sodium). Electrolyte abnormalities can lead to conduction abnormalities in the heart and lead to cardiac arrhythmia; meaning that you can develop incredibly dangerous abnormal heart rhythms.

Avoidance of diuretics outside of a supervised medical setting is strongly advised.

3.1 Furosemide (Lasix)
Description: Furosemide is a loop diuretic used to reduce fluid accumulation. It is commonly used to treat excess edema from heart failure.

Side Effects:
- **Electrolyte Imbalance**: Can cause deficiencies in potassium, sodium, and magnesium.
- **Dehydration**: Risk of severe dehydration and reduced blood pressure.
- **Kidney Damage**: Impairment of kidney function can occur even from short term use.

3.2 Hydrochlorothiazide (HCTZ)
Description: HCTZ is a thiazide diuretic used to manage fluid retention and hypertension.

Side Effects:
- **Electrolyte Imbalance**: Similar to furosemide, it can cause imbalances in potassium and sodium.
- **Dehydration**: Potential for dehydration and low blood pressure.
- **Gout**: Increased risk of gout due to elevated uric acid levels.

4. Stimulants
Stimulants are used to enhance energy, focus, and endurance. They work by increasing the release of neurotransmitters like dopamine and norepinephrine.

4.1 Ephedrine

Description: Ephedrine is used to increase metabolism and promote fat loss. It is a potent stimulant with a half-life of approximately 3-6 hours. This used to be a widely popular stimulant in the 1980s-1990s and 2000s and has since become less available due to the risks and less widely used.

Side Effects:
- **Increased Heart Rate**: Risk of tachycardia and palpitations, and dangerous heart rhythms
- **High Blood Pressure**: Risk of hypertension.
- **Insomnia**: Difficulty sleeping due to stimulating effects.
- **Anxiety**: Potential for increased anxiety and agitation.

4.2 Caffeine

Description: Caffeine is widely used to enhance alertness and physical performance and is perhaps the most common drug used worldwide. It has a half-life of approximately 3-5 hours. The only medical use for caffeine is generally in the neonatal ICU setting for managing respiratory failure in neonates and post lumbar puncture headaches. Off-label, it can be used for the treatment of certain headaches such as tension headache or post spinal tap headaches. There has also been a correlation made between caffeine intake and the reduction of fat content in the liver, though notably most often studied with black coffee only. Caffeine's benefits and side effects exist alongside a spectrum with higher doses posing a risk of more adverse effects.

Side Effects:
- **Insomnia**: Common side effect, especially if taken later in the day.
- **Nervousness**: Potential for increased anxiety and jitteriness.
- **Digestive Issues**: Can cause stomach upset or acid reflux.
- **Heart Palpitations**: Risk of irregular heartbeats.

4.3 Clenbuterol

Description: Clenbuterol is a beta-2 agonist used for its fat-burning properties. It is in the same family as the common asthma/COPD inhaler; albuterol (in USA) and salbutamol (in Canada). It has a half-life of approximately 36-48 hours. It is not approved in Canada or USA for any medical purposes. Clenbuterol has been linked to cases of sudden cardiac death. It leads to significant tachycardia while simultaneously depleting potassium levels, which is a very dangerous combination.

Side Effects:
- **Tachycardia**: Increased heart rate and risk of arrhythmias.
- **Tremors**: Muscle shaking or tremors.
- **Insomnia**: Difficulty sleeping.
- **Electrolyte Imbalance**: Risk of hypokalemia (low potassium levels) which can lead to abnormal heart rhythms.

4.4 Methylhexanamine (DMAA)

Description: Perhaps the most infamous pre-workout ingredient that was used in numerous well known pre-workout supplements in the 2010s. This ingredient has been sold under various names (ex. Geranium extract) and has since been banned in some countries and by most sports authorities.

Side Effects:
- **Tachycardia**: Increased heart rate and risk of arrhythmias.
- **Tremors**: Muscle shaking or tremors.
- **Insomnia**

4.5 Yohimbine

Description: Another formerly popular pre-workout ingredient that was used for its stimulant properties. Other advertised benefits included the treatment of erectile dysfunction and low libido.

Side Effects:

- **Tachycardia**: Increased heart rate and risk of arrhythmias and hypertension
- **Tremors**: Muscle shaking or tremors were commonly noted

Doctor's comment: DMAA, yohimbine, clenbuterol and ephedrine are all genuinely dangerous drugs and can lead to sudden death.

5. Erythropoietin (EPO)
EPO is a hormone that stimulates red blood cell production. It is used to enhance endurance by increasing the oxygen-carrying capacity of the blood.

5.1 Recombinant EPO
Description: Recombinant EPO is a synthetic version of the hormone used to treat certain types of anemia, but it is also abused for its performance-enhancing effects.

Side Effects:
- **Increased Blood Viscosity**: Risk of blood clots and stroke due to thicker blood.
- **Hypertension**: Elevated blood pressure.
- **Headaches**: Common side effect.
- **Flu-like Symptoms**: Fever, fatigue, and muscle aches.

Doctor's comment: Anabolic steroids and testosterone all increase EPO, which is why they cause a high hemoglobin and hematocrit.

6. Thyroid Hormones
Thyroid hormones, such as T3 (liothyronine) and T4 (levothyroxine), are synthetic versions of the naturally occurring hormones produced by the thyroid gland. These hormones regulate the body's metabolism energy production, and protein synthesis. In the fitness and bodybuilding community, thyroid hormones are used for their ability to significantly enhance metabolic rate, leading to increased fat loss and improved energy expenditure. T3 is the more potent form, acting quickly to increase metabolic activity, while T4 is converted into T3

within the body at a slower rate. Typically, individuals who use thyroid hormones do so during cutting phases to achieve a leaner physique while maintaining muscle mass. They are often used in conjunction with other performance-enhancing drugs, such as anabolic steroids, to offset the potential muscle loss that can occur during calorie deficits.

Although thyroid hormones can accelerate fat loss and improve overall energy levels, they come with significant risks. Excessive use can lead to thyroid dysfunction, where the body's natural thyroid hormone production is suppressed, leading to a dependency on synthetic hormones. Users may also experience symptoms of hyperthyroidism, such as rapid heart rate, anxiety, excessive sweating, and muscle weakness. If dosing is improperly managed, the risks include cardiac issues such as arrhythmias or even potential heart failure due to the overstimulation of metabolic activity. Additionally, thyroid hormone use can lead to bone density loss over time, increasing the risk of fractures. Post-use, users often experience a rebound effect, where their metabolism slows significantly due to the suppression of natural thyroid function, which can make weight maintenance challenging.

Doctor's comment: Use of thyroid hormones without a medical reason can lead to atrial fibrillation and also heart failure.

7. Nootropics

Nootropics, often referred to as "smart drugs," are a class of substances used to enhance cognitive functions such as focus, memory, and overall mental performance. In the fitness and wellness community, nootropics are frequently utilized for their ability to improve focus during training sessions, enhance motivation, and support faster learning of new skills or techniques. Compounds such as modafinil, phenylpiracetam, and alpha-GPC are some of the more popular nootropics, each working through different mechanisms to influence neurotransmitters such as ldopamine, acetylcholine, and norepinephrine. Despite their perceived benefits, nootropics come with their own set of risks, including potential for addiction, disrupted sleep patterns, and increased anxiety. The use of these substances should be approached cautiously, as their long-term effects on brain health are still not fully understood.

7.1 Modafinil

Description: Modafinil is a wakefulness-promoting agent commonly used for its ability to enhance alertness, focus, and cognitive performance. It is often prescribed for narcolepsy and sleep disorders but has found use in the fitness and productivity community for its cognitive-enhancing effects. The evidence supporting modafinil as a nootropic is relatively strong, with numerous studies demonstrating improvements in attention, executive function, and working memory. However, while modafinil is generally considered safe, it is not without side effects, which may include headaches, anxiety, and, in some cases, cardiovascular risks. Its long-term safety profile is still under investigation, and caution is advised for those considering its use. It is often banned by sporting authorities and should only be used with a prescription.

7.2 Phenylpiracetam

Description: Phenylpiracetam is a derivative of piracetam, designed to be more potent and effective in enhancing memory, learning capacity, and physical stamina. The evidence for phenylpiracetam's efficacy is mixed; while animal studies have shown improvements in cognitive function and endurance, there is limited scientific research on humans to substantiate these claims. Some users report enhanced focus and reduced mental fatigue, but the data remains largely anecdotal. Side effects are typically mild but can include headaches, irritability, and sleep disturbances. The lack of robust clinical trials raises questions about both its efficacy and safety in the long term.

7.3 Noopept

Description: Noopept is a synthetic nootropic similar in function to racetams, commonly used for improving memory and learning capacity. It is believed to enhance cognitive performance by increasing nerve growth factor and brain-derived neurotrophic factor levels. Some animal studies suggest potential benefits for neuroprotection and cognitive enhancement, but human research is scarce and of variable quality. While it is considered probably safe, side effects such as headaches, irritability, and nausea have been reported. More rigorous human studies are needed to establish its effectiveness and safety profile conclusively.

7.4 Alpha-GPC

Description: Alpha-GPC is a choline compound that acts as a precursor to acetylcholine, a neurotransmitter associated with memory and learning. It is used as a nootropic to improve mental clarity, cognitive function, and focus. Evidence for Alpha-GPC's effectiveness is quite reasonable, especially in older adults, with studies showing improvements in memory and attention. It is also used in athletic contexts for its potential to increase power output. Side effects are generally minimal but can include gastrointestinal discomfort and headaches. The quality of the evidence is moderate, with a need for more extensive, placebo-controlled studies before it even approaches official medical use.

7.5 L-Theanine

Description: L-Theanine is an amino acid commonly found in green tea, known for promoting relaxation without causing drowsiness. It is often used in combination with caffeine to enhance focus and reduce the jitteriness associated with caffeine intake. The evidence supporting L-theanine is solid, with several studies demonstrating its efficacy in reducing stress and promoting a state of relaxed alertness. It has an excellent safety profile, with minimal reported side effects, making it one of the most commonly recommended nootropics for beginners from online communities. However, more long-term studies would further solidify its role in cognitive enhancement. Currently, there is no formal medical indication for its use.

7.6 Bacopa Monnieri

Description: Bacopa Monnieri is an adaptogenic herb traditionally used in Ayurvedic medicine for its cognitive-enhancing properties. It is believed to improve memory and reduce anxiety by increasing serotonin and reducing oxidative stress in the brain. Evidence for Bacopa Monnieri exists but is variable, with several studies showing improvements in memory and cognitive performance, particularly after prolonged use of eight weeks or more. However, there are no robust long-term trials. Side effects can include gastrointestinal discomfort, nausea, and increased bowel movements. Although it has a good safety profile based on what is known at this time, the full extent of its long-term efficacy requires more in-depth research.

7.7 Rhodiola Rosea

Description: Rhodiola Rosea is an adaptogenic herb used to reduce fatigue, enhance mood, and improve cognitive function. It is believed to work by reducing cortisol levels and increasing resilience to stress. The evidence supporting Rhodiola is moderate, with multiple studies indicating improvements in fatigue, anxiety, and overall cognitive function, particularly in high-stress situations. Side effects are minimal, typically involving mild gastrointestinal issues or dizziness. However, variability in the quality of commercial supplements and a lack of long-term studies are potential limitations in evaluating its efficacy and safety.

7.8 Lion's Mane Mushroom

Description: Lion's Mane Mushroom is a medicinal mushroom used for its potential to promote neurogenesis and improve cognitive function. It is thought to stimulate the production of nerve growth factor, which may support brain health and memory. The evidence is promising but still limited, with a few human studies suggesting potential improvements in mild cognitive impairment and anxiety. Lion's Mane is generally considered safe, with side effects rarely reported, though some users experience gastrointestinal discomfort. While the early findings are encouraging, more rigorous, long-term studies are needed to verify its cognitive-enhancing effects and safety profile.

Doctor's comment: It is difficult to know whether nootropics actually work or largely induce placebo effects. Measuring cognitive performance is difficult for obvious reasons. While nootropics do show some promise for playing a role in the future for those with early dementia, it is unlikely they truly have a significant effect beyond placebo for young people.

Conclusion

Performance-enhancing drugs encompass a broad range of substances beyond anabolic steroids, each with distinct mechanisms, dosages, and side effects. Selective androgen receptor modulators (SARMs) such as Ostarine, Ligandrol, Andarine, Cardarine, and YK-11 offer varying risks. Peptide hormones such as HGH, insulin, and IGF-1 provide muscle growth and recovery but come with their own set of potential side effects. Diuretics such as furosemide and hydrochlorothiazide are used to manipulate fluid levels, while stimulants such as ephedrine, caffeine, and clenbuterol enhance energy and performance. Erythropoietin (EPO) boosts endurance but can lead to serious cardiovascular risks.

In conclusion, many drugs exist for performance enhancement, whether the goal is physical enhancement or cognitive enhancement (in the case of nootropics). Although, almost all compounds discussed in this chapter are banned for competitive athletes. The best approach to PED use is skepticism, given that we currently lack robust placebo-controlled trials and cannot draw any definitive conclusions on these compounds.

Chapter 20: Supplements

Throughout the latter parts of the 1990s, supplements began to gain enormous popularity in the fitness industry. By the 2010s, they were used by people from all walks of life. From vitamins to protein supplements and various herbal brands, different supplements marketed for various purposes exist on the market today. The goal of this chapter is to review some common and less common supplements, while also providing an opinion on each one.

Whey Protein
- **Description:** A high-quality protein derived from milk, quickly absorbed by the body.
- **Benefits:** Supports muscle recovery, promotes muscle growth, and aids in meeting daily protein needs.
- **Side Effects:** Generally safe, but some types may cause digestive issues in lactose-intolerant individuals.

Opinion: One of the most common supplements used globally and one of the most useful ones anyone can take. While it doesn't have any direct performance enhancing benefits, it helps you meet your protein intake goals.

Creatine Monohydrate
- **Description:** A naturally occurring compound found in small amounts in certain foods, such as red meat, and synthesized in the body.
- **Benefits:** Enhances strength, increases lean muscle mass, and improves exercise performance, especially in high-intensity activities.
- **Side Effects:** May cause water retention and gastrointestinal discomfort in some individuals. Also, may not work in some users.

Opinion: A very common supplement and one of the few performance-enhancing supplements that actually works. Long term data has not raised any safety concerns. As a side note, it does not directly raise your serum creatinine levels on blood tests, which is very important for healthcare professionals to know.

Branched-Chain Amino Acids (BCAAs)
- **Description:** Composed of three essential amino acids: leucine, isoleucine, and valine.
- **Benefits:** Theoretical benefits include increased muscle protein synthesis, reduced muscle soreness, and decreases exercise-induced fatigue.
- **Side Effects:** No evidence-based safety concerns.

Opinion: BCAAs have no direct benefits on their own in a user that already meets their protein intake targets.

Beta-Alanine
- **Description:** A non-essential amino acid that helps produce carnosine, which buffers acid in muscles.
- **Benefits:** Increases endurance and performance in high-intensity exercises by delaying muscle fatigue.
- **Side Effects:** It causes a tingling or flushing sensations which can be unpleasant for some.

Opinion: Likely useful to some marginal extent for endurance-based performances but unlikely to provide much benefit for others.

D-aspartic acid (DAA)
- **Description:** A non-essential amino acid that stimulates LH levels to rise and thereby, in theory, increases endogenous testosterone production.
- **Benefits:** Studies did show a mild increase in LH levels which were transient, lasting about 3 weeks. Testosterone levels also climbed during that time but then dropped back down to baseline.
- **Side Effects:** Some users experience gastrointestinal upset.

Opinion: On paper this supplement looks great. It is a supplement that can cause your body to make more testosterone – at least, in theory. In real life, it is one of those interventions that does not translate over to any true difference in performance. This is generally true for all testosterone booster supplements. It may play a theoretical role for those who want to stop steroids or TRT and restart their natural testosterone production. However, this needs to be studied before it can be recommended.

Fish Oil (Omega-3 Fatty Acids)
- **Description:** Derived from fish, rich in omega-3 fatty acids (EPA and DHA).
- **Benefits:** Reduces inflammation, supports heart health, and may aid in recovery from exercise.
- **Side Effects:** High doses can lead to digestive issues and an increased risk of bleeding.

Opinion: It can be a good supplement for many users, but the evidence in recent years has shown mixed data. There may even be a risk of atrial fibrillation.

Caffeine
- **Description:** A central nervous system stimulant commonly found in coffee, tea, and supplements.
- **Benefits:** Enhances focus, energy, and performance; may improve endurance and reduce perceived exertion. Medical indications were mentioned earlier in the book.
- **Side Effects:** Can cause jitters, insomnia, increased heart rate, and digestive issues in sensitive individuals or in high doses.

Opinion: The most powerful and legal performance enhancing agent is caffeine.

Glutamine
- **Description:** An amino acid that plays a key role in muscle recovery and immune function.

- **Benefits:** In theory, it supports muscle recovery, immune health, and gut health, especially after intense training.
- **Side Effects:** Generally safe, but high doses may lead to gastrointestinal discomfort.

Opinion: Unlikely to be of significant benefit for most people.

Multivitamins
- **Description:** Supplements that contain a combination of vitamins and minerals.
- **Benefits:** Helps fill nutritional gaps and supports overall health, particularly for those with limited diets.
- **Side Effects:** Overconsumption of certain vitamins and minerals can lead to silent side effects.

Opinion: Useful for those who do not have balanced diets, but not useful for those who do have balanced diets.

ZMA (Zinc, Magnesium Aspartate, and Vitamin B6)
- **Description:** A combination supplement often marketed for athletes.
- **Benefits:** Supports recovery, enhances sleep quality, and may improve hormonal balance in theory.
- **Side Effects:** Generally well-tolerated; high doses of zinc can cause nausea and interfere with copper absorption. However, the copper issue only occurs at prolonged high doses of zinc supplementation and is not nearly as common as most think.

Opinion: Anecdotally, it has been reported to be useful for sleep. Those without zinc deficiency are unlikely to see an increase in their testosterone levels.

L-Carnitine
- **Description:** An amino acid derivative involved in fat metabolism.
- **Benefits:** May enhance fat burning, improve exercise performance, and support recovery.

- **Side Effects:** Some individuals may experience gastrointestinal upset or a fishy body odor. Can potentially lead to coronary artery disease due to increasing TMAO levels.

Opinion: There is contradictory data on L-carnitine and whether it increases the risk of heart disease. It can increase TMAO and has been correlated to increased atherosclerosis and carotid plaque buildup. It is best to exercise caution with this one and probably avoid it.

L-Arginine
- **Description:** An amino acid that serves as a precursor to nitric oxide.
- **Benefits:** May improve blood flow, enhance exercise performance, and support recovery by promoting vasodilation.
- **Side Effects:** Can cause gastrointestinal discomfort.

Opinion: There is generally no noticeable benefit to supplementing arginine.

Rhodiola Rosea
- **Description:** An adaptogenic herb known for its potential stress-reducing properties.
- **Benefits:** May improve endurance, reduce fatigue, and enhance mental performance, especially under stress. These are anecdotal benefits.
- **Side Effects:** Generally well-tolerated acutely; some may experience dry mouth or dizziness.

Opinion: The evidence is generally weak for any noticeable performance benefits.

Ashwagandha
- **Description:** An adaptogenic herb used in Ayurvedic medicine.
- **Benefits:** May reduce stress, improve mood, enhance physical performance, and support muscle strength.
- **Side Effects:** Generally safe, but some individuals may experience gastrointestinal upset or drowsiness.

Opinion: Those with thyroid disorders should be cautious, as recommended by companies selling ashwagandha supplements. This is thought to be due to increased T3 and T4 levels, which makes it harmful in those with hyperthyroidism. There has been evidence showing that it can be a useful supplement for some athletes.

Vitamin D
- **Description:** A fat-soluble vitamin important for bone health and immune function.
- **Benefits:** Supports calcium absorption, may improve mood, and is essential for muscle function. Possible benefits for cancer, hypertension, dementia and heart disease prevention.
- **Side Effects:** Excessive intake can lead to toxicity, causing nausea, weakness, and kidney problems. Although, toxicity is relatively rare.

Opinion: The most famous supplement of the 21st century. While the evidence supporting its use has been all over the spectrum, it is generally recognized that maintaining a healthy vitamin D level is likely better than being deficient. While vitamin D is quite likely to be a very useful supplement, it may also be a negative inflammatory biomarker. That means that deficiency could be a sign of relatively poor health rather than an actual cause for illness. However, there is still some data showing benefits at optimal levels in contrast to deficiency. Therefore, supplementation to maintain a normal level is recommended.

Coenzyme Q10 (CoQ10)
- **Description:** An antioxidant that plays a crucial role in energy production in cells.
- **Benefits:** May enhance exercise performance, support heart health, and reduce oxidative stress. Many of these reported benefits have not been replicated in studies.
- **Side Effects:** Generally well-tolerated; high doses may cause gastrointestinal issues.

Opinion: The evidence supporting its benefits is relatively weak. It was previously used alongside statin therapy to see if it would help offset the side effects of statin, since, in theory, statin use leads to depletion of coenzyme q10. Unfortunately, this supplementation was shown to be unsuccessful in offsetting the side effects.

Probiotics
- **Description:** Live microorganisms that can provide health benefits when consumed in adequate amounts.
- **Benefits:** Support gut health, improve digestion, and may enhance immune function.
- **Side Effects:** Generally safe; some individuals may experience mild digestive discomfort initially.

Opinion: There are many studied health benefits with probiotics, though, it is important not to have very high expectations. It is possible that prebiotics and postbiotics offer even more benefits than probiotics.

Curcumin (Turmeric Extract)
- **Description:** The active compound in turmeric with anti-inflammatory properties.
- **Benefits:** May reduce inflammation, support joint health, and improve recovery after exercise.
- **Side Effects:** Generally safe; high doses may cause gastrointestinal upset.

Opinion: Turmeric does not absorb well, especially if taken without food or alongside antacids.

Green Tea Extract
- **Description:** Concentrated form of green tea rich in antioxidants, particularly catechins.
- **Benefits:** May support fat loss, enhance metabolism, and improve exercise performance.
- **Side Effects:** High doses may lead to liver toxicity and gastrointestinal discomfort in sensitive individuals.

Opinion: This is one of the few supplements that has been implicated in cases of severe liver failure.

Citrulline Malate
- **Description:** A compound combining citrulline (an amino acid) and malate (a compound involved in energy production).
- **Benefits:** May improve endurance, reduce fatigue, and enhance recovery by increasing nitric oxide levels.
- **Side Effects:** Generally well-tolerated; some may experience gastrointestinal discomfort.

Opinion: Potentially a useful supplement for cosmetic reasons, without any known safety concerns. It can lead to a "vascular" appearance in some.

Glucosamine, Chondroitin and MSM
- **Description:** Compounds often taken together to support joint health.
- **Benefits:** Glucosamine is involved in the formation of cartilage, while chondroitin helps retain water in the cartilage. They may reduce joint pain and improve mobility, particularly in osteoarthritis.
- **Side Effects:** Generally safe but can cause digestive issues in some individuals.

Opinion: The evidence is generally weak in terms of its efficacy, with most utility being seen for osteoarthritis pain management only. It does not reverse osteoarthritis itself.

Fibre Supplements
- **Description:** Supplements such as psyllium husk or inulin, which are used to increase dietary fibre intake.
- **Benefits:** Supports digestive health and regular bowel movements, may help with weight management by promoting satiety. It can also improve cholesterol levels.
- **Side Effects:** Some may experience bloating or gas, especially with abrupt increases in fibre.

Opinion: For those unable to obtain fibre from dietary sources, the use of fibre supplements is highly recommended due to the many health benefits of fibre. Although, high fibre intake is not necessarily ideal for everyone. Users should also gradually increase their fibre intake and not abruptly initiate high intake.

HMB (Beta-Hydroxy Beta-Methylbutyrate)
- **Description:** A metabolite of the amino acid leucine, which is a biological switch in the body that activates protein synthesis.
- **Benefits:** Thought to reduce muscle breakdown during intense exercise and enhance muscle growth and recovery.
- **Side Effects:** Generally well-tolerated, but high doses could cause gastrointestinal discomfort.

Opinion: Caution should be taken as HMB supplements, at times, may contain heavy metals.

Collagen Peptides
- **Description:** Derived from animal connective tissues.
- **Benefits:** Often taken to support skin, joint, and bone health; in theory it would improve skin elasticity and hydration and, theoretically, could reduce joint pain.
- **Side Effects:** Generally considered safe, but some individuals may experience digestive issues.

Opinion: There is no robust evidence supporting its efficacy.

Alpha-Lipoic Acid (ALA)
- **Description:** An antioxidant that plays a role in energy metabolism.
- **Benefits:** May help reduce oxidative stress, support weight management, and improve insulin sensitivity.
- **Side Effects:** While generally considered safe, high doses may lead to gastrointestinal discomfort.

Opinion (and fact): Not to be confused with alpha linolenic acid which is an omega 3 fatty acid.

L-Theanine
- **Description:** An amino acid found primarily in tea leaves.
- **Benefits:** Known for promoting relaxation without drowsiness, may improve focus and cognitive performance, particularly when combined with caffeine.
- **Side Effects:** Generally well-tolerated and considered safe for most people.

Opinion: It may have utility if combined with caffeine.

Fenugreek
- **Description:** An herb often used for its potential health benefits.
- **Benefits:** May support healthy blood sugar levels, enhance libido, and promote muscle growth.
- **Side Effects:** While generally considered safe, some may experience gastrointestinal discomfort or allergic reactions.

Opinion: There is limited evidence supporting its efficacy.

L-Carnitine Tartrate
- **Description:** A form of L-carnitine that may improve exercise performance.
- **Benefits:** Supports fat metabolism and may reduce muscle soreness after exercise.
- **Side Effects:** Generally considered safe acutely; high doses may cause gastrointestinal discomfort or a fishy odor. Long-term, it may pose a risk of developing atherosclerosis.

Opinion: Like all carnitine supplements, it could raise levels of trimethylamine N-oxide (TMAO) in the body which can lead to atherosclerosis and subsequent coronary artery disease.

N-Acetyl Cysteine (NAC)
- **Description:** A supplement form of cysteine, an amino acid. It is also used for the treatment of Tylenol overdose.
- **Benefits:** Acts as an antioxidant, supports detoxification, and may improve respiratory health.

- **Side Effects:** While generally safe, some may experience nausea or gastrointestinal upset.

Opinion: It has theoretical benefits as well as mainstream medical efficacy for treating Tylenol overdose. Some newer medical indications include the treatment of acute liver failure. It has also been studied for the treatment of fatty liver, with mixed results.

Chia Seeds
- **Description:** Tiny seeds rich in nutrients, including omega-3 fatty acids and fiber.
- **Benefits:** May promote digestive health, support heart health, and enhance satiety.
- **Side Effects:** Generally safe; excessive intake may lead to digestive issues if not consumed with adequate water.

Opinion: A good source of plant-based omega-3 fatty acids.

Spirulina
- **Description:** A blue-green algae known for its nutrient density.
- **Benefits:** May boost energy levels, support immune function, and provide a rich source of antioxidants.
- **Side Effects:** Generally safe; some may experience digestive upset or allergic reactions.

Opinion: Unlikely to be of any benefit.

Resveratrol
- **Description:** A polyphenol found in red wine, grapes, and berries.
- **Benefits:** May have antioxidant properties, support heart health, and promote longevity. Some anti-cancer benefits as well.
- **Side Effects:** While generally safe, high doses could interact with blood-thinning medications.

Opinion: There is a lot of evidence supporting its benefits, but it is generally considered best to consume it from dietary sources instead of pills. Many nutrients are beneficial but only truly useful when consumed within food rather than pills. The reason is that supplement manufacturing can never guarantee retention of bioavailability.

Vitamin C
- **Description:** An essential vitamin and powerful antioxidant.
- **Benefits:** Supports immune function, aids in collagen synthesis, and promotes skin health.
- **Side Effects:** While generally safe, excessive intake may cause gastrointestinal upset or diarrhea.

Opinion: If your diet does not have sufficient fruits and vegetables, then supplementing vitamin C is necessary. If the diet is well balanced with adequate caloric intake, then your vitamin C intake is likely to be sufficient.

Vitamin A
- **Description:** A fat-soluble vitamin essential for vision, immune function, and skin health.
- **Benefits:** Supports eye health, particularly in preventing night blindness; helps with immune function and skin cell turnover.
- **Formulations:** Retinol (from animal sources) and beta-carotene (from plant sources).
- **Side Effects:** Excessive intake, particularly of retinol, can cause toxicity leading to liver damage, dry skin, and blurred vision.

Opinion: It is best to consume vitamin A via dietary sources and most people should not take vitamin A supplements.

B-Complex Vitamins
- **Description:** A group of eight water-soluble vitamins (B1, B2, B3, B5, B6, B7, B9, and B12) that play vital roles in metabolism, energy production, and nervous system health.
- **Benefits:** Supports energy levels, metabolism, brain function, and the formation of red blood cells.

- **Formulations:** Available as individual B vitamins (e.g., B12 as methylcobalamin or cyanocobalamin) or as B-complex supplements containing all eight.
- **Side Effects:** Generally safe; high doses of some B vitamins, such as B6, may cause nerve damage over time.

Opinion: Most people do not need these but, anecdotally, it may help athletes and recreational lifters who spend very long hours training. In other words, it could be useful for those who do very extended periods of intense training. B12 supplements in isolation are unlikely to offer any benefit beyond the scope of this.

Vitamin E
- **Description:** A fat-soluble antioxidant that helps protect cells from oxidative damage.
- **Benefits:** Supports immune function, skin health, and prevents damage to cells from free radicals. It helps to treat fatty liver disease as well.
- **Formulations:** Tocopherols and tocotrienols, with alpha-tocopherol being the most common form in supplements.
- **Side Effects:** Excessive intake can interfere with blood clotting and increase the risk of bleeding.

Opinion: The main indication is for fatty liver disease with F2 stage fibrosis. Vitamin E supplements have been correlated with an increase of all-cause mortality as well as some cancers. Generally, it is best to avoid casual use of this supplement.

Vitamin K
- **Description:** A fat-soluble vitamin important for blood clotting and bone health.
- **Benefits:** Helps in the synthesis of proteins needed for blood clotting; supports bone health by regulating calcium.
- **Formulations:** Vitamin K1 (phylloquinone, found in leafy greens) and K2 (menaquinone, found in animal products and fermented foods).

- **Side Effects:** Generally safe, however it can interact with blood-thinning medications such as warfarin. Individuals who use blood thinners should not use any vitamin K.

Opinion: K2 supplements have shown a lot of promise in recent years. They may help reduce arterial calcification and lower the risk of coronary artery disease. More studies are needed but this is probably one of the most promising supplements on the market.

Boron
- **Description:** A trace mineral found in various foods and supplements.
- **Benefits:** May support bone health, enhance testosterone levels, and improve cognitive function.
- **Side Effects:** Generally safe at recommended doses; excessive intake can lead to toxicity.

Opinion: Often marketed as a testosterone booster but, similarly to other testosterone boosters, is unlikely to yield any noticeable effects. It may increase the number to some extent, but it's unlikely that anything noticeable happens in terms of clinical effect.

Selenium
- **Description:** A trace mineral that acts as an antioxidant and plays a role in thyroid function.
- **Benefits:** Supports immune function, promotes thyroid hormone metabolism, and protects cells from oxidative stress.
- **Formulations:** Selenomethionine and sodium selenite are common supplement forms.
- **Side Effects:** Excessive intake can cause selenosis, leading to hair loss, fatigue, and digestive upset.

Opinion: Most people do not require selenium supplements.

Zinc
- **Description:** An essential mineral involved in immune function, wound healing, and DNA synthesis.

- **Benefits:** Supports immune health, promotes wound healing, and aids in taste and smell functions.
- **Formulations:** Zinc citrate, zinc gluconate, and zinc picolinate are common forms used in supplements.
- **Side Effects:** High doses may cause nausea, vomiting, and interfere with the absorption of other minerals, such as copper.

Opinion: There could be some limited use benefit for high level athletes. However, for most people, supplementation is unlikely to be of any benefit. While zinc has been studied for immune system function, the findings are controversial. It is largely zinc lozenges that are perhaps useful for throat infections, rather than zinc intake itself.

Calcium
- **Description:** A crucial mineral for bone health, muscle function, and nerve transmission.
- **Benefits:** Promotes strong bones and teeth, supports heart health, and aids in muscle contraction.
- **Formulations:** Calcium carbonate (most common, but requires stomach acid for absorption), calcium citrate (easier to absorb, especially in older adults), and calcium lactate.
- **Side Effects:** Excessive intake can lead to kidney stones, constipation, and interference with the absorption of other minerals.

Opinion: Given possible links to the development of coronary artery disease, it is best to limit this supplement to using it only when recommended by a doctor.

Magnesium
- **Description:** An essential mineral involved in over 300 biochemical reactions in the body.
- **Benefits:** Supports muscle relaxation, nervous system health, and helps regulate blood sugar and blood pressure.
- **Formulations:** Magnesium citrate (largely for relieving constipation), magnesium glycinate (for relaxation and sleep),

magnesium oxide (higher concentration but less bioavailable), and magnesium malate.
- **Side Effects:** High doses can lead to diarrhea, nausea, and abdominal cramping.

Opinion: It is important to double check the formulation that you are using; magnesium citrate can cause diarrhea whereas magnesium oxide is difficult to absorb. Magnesium glycinate is the most useful formulation.

Ginger
- **Description:** A root widely used for its medicinal properties, particularly in digestive and anti-inflammatory support.
- **Benefits:** Helps reduce nausea, supports digestion, and may have anti-inflammatory effects.
- **Formulations:** Fresh ginger, ginger extract, and powdered ginger supplements.
- **Side Effects:** Generally safe; excessive intake may cause heartburn or gastrointestinal discomfort, but this is dependent on the supplement formulation.

Opinion: A good treatment option for mild nausea and indigestion.

Garlic
- **Description:** A popular herb used both in cooking and as a supplement for its health benefits, particularly cardiovascular.
- **Benefits:** May lower blood pressure, improve cholesterol levels, and support immune function.
- **Formulations:** Fresh garlic, garlic oil, and aged garlic extract (odorless formulations available).
- **Side Effects:** Can cause bad breath, digestive upset, or an allergic reaction in sensitive individuals.

Opinion: The lipid profile benefits of garlic supplementation are quite limited and not sufficient enough to make garlic a widely recommended supplement.

Betaine Anhydrous
- **Description:** A naturally occurring compound derived from choline. Betaine is found in foods such as beets, spinach, and whole grains. Betaine is used as a supplement for its potential to enhance athletic performance, improve body composition, and support heart and liver health through its role in methylation processes. These are the descriptive and hypothetical benefits, but the literature is mixed, and its benefits not that well studied.
- **Benefits:** May improve strength and power during exercise based on weak evidence. It may also reduce homocysteine levels; homocysteine is considered a cardiac risk factor. Emerging research also suggests a potential role in reducing fat accumulation in the liver.
- **Formulations:** Available as a standalone powder or in combination with pre-workout or post-workout supplements. Often found in supplement products in dosages of 2.5 grams per day.
- **Side Effects:** Generally well-tolerated, but can cause mild gastrointestinal discomfort in some individuals, particularly when taken in higher doses.

Opinion: It might be a useful supplement, but its performance benefits are not well understood yet.

Chapter 21: A Closer Look at Creatine

As one of the most common supplements in the past few decades, creatine deserves its own chapter.

Creatine: An Overview
Creatine is a naturally occurring compound found in the body, primarily in skeletal muscle, where it plays a critical role in energy production during high-intensity exercise. Structurally, creatine is a nitrogenous organic acid synthesized from the amino acids glycine, arginine, and methionine, with most of it being stored as phosphocreatine. This stored form serves as a rapid energy reserve, facilitating the regeneration of adenosine triphosphate (ATP) which is the body's primary energy currency. Creatine's ability to support rapid energy production is what makes it popular amongst strength and power athletes.

The History of Creatine
The discovery of creatine goes back to the 19th century when it was identified in meat product extracts. In 1832, a French scientist name Michel Eugène Chevreul first isolated creatine from skeletal muscle, naming it after the Greek word "kreas," which meant meat. By the early 20th century, researchers began to understand its role in energy metabolism. However, creatine's emergence as a sports supplement did not occur until the 1990s, following studies demonstrating its effectiveness in improving athletic performance. During this time, athletes at the 1992 Barcelona Olympics popularized creatine supplementation, which started the widespread use of creatine supplements.

Dosing and Supplementation
Creatine supplementation traditionally began with a "loading" phase which entailed the consumption of 20 grams per day, divided into 4-5 doses, over five to seven days; this strategy would be beneficial to saturate muscle creatine stores. After the loading phase, a maintenance dose of 3-5 grams daily sustains these elevated levels. For those who

preferred to avoid loading, consuming 3-5 grams daily from the outset was also noted to achieve saturation.

Today, we know that there is no real benefit to loading creatine; taking 5g daily is optimal. Creatine is most effective when taken with carbohydrate-rich meals, as insulin spikes enhance creatine uptake by muscle cells.

The Science Behind Creatine's Benefits
The primary mechanism through which creatine enhances performance is its role in the phosphocreatine energy system. During short bursts of high-intensity activity, ATP is rapidly depleted and must be regenerated. Phosphocreatine donates a phosphate group to adenosine diphosphate (ADP), replenishing ATP stores and enabling sustained performance. By increasing phosphocreatine availability, creatine allows athletes to perform more repetitions, sprint faster, or lift heavier weights, ultimately leading to greater training adaptations over time. Beyond energy production, creatine has been shown to promote cell volumization (muscle hydration) and influence signaling pathways that support muscle growth. Therefore, the realized benefits of creatine have evolved to also support hypertrophy.

Benefits of Creatine Supplementation
Creatine's benefits extend beyond athletic performance. In addition to improving strength, power, and endurance during high-intensity activities, creatine supports muscle hypertrophy by enhancing training volume and reducing fatigue. Emerging research also highlights its potential cognitive benefits, particularly in aging populations or individuals with neurological conditions. Creatine may improve memory, processing speed, and brain energy metabolism. However, more research is needed before it can be recommended for any medical purposes.

Use in Sports
Creatine's role in sports performance has been extensively validated, making it one of the most researched ergogenic aids available. It is

particularly beneficial for athletes engaged in anaerobic or high-intensity sports, such as weightlifting, sprinting, or football. Studies consistently demonstrate improvements in strength, power, and exercise capacity with creatine supplementation. For endurance athletes, the benefits are less pronounced but may still include enhanced performance during sprint intervals or resistance training. Creatine is not banned by major sporting organizations, making it a legal and widely accepted supplement for competitive athletes.

Safety of Creatine
Despite misconceptions about its safety, creatine is one of the safest dietary supplements available. Long-term studies involving doses of up to 20 grams per day have found no adverse effects on kidney or liver function in healthy individuals. The most common side effect is temporary water retention, which increases body weight. However, it is important to mention that not every user experiences water retention. Mild gastrointestinal discomfort can occur, particularly with higher doses, but this is often mitigated by splitting doses throughout the day. While individuals with pre-existing kidney issues should consult a physician before supplementation, creatine is considered safe for the vast majority of users.

Types of Creatine
Creatine monohydrate is the most researched and widely used form, known for its safety, efficacy, and affordability. It is highly bioavailable, meaning the body can efficiently absorb and utilize it. Other forms, such as creatine hydrochloride and buffered creatine (Kre-Alkalyn), claim to offer advantages like reduced bloating or improved absorption, but these claims lack robust scientific backing. Studies comparing different forms consistently show that creatine monohydrate performs as well or better than newer, more expensive formulations.

Creatine Monohydrate vs. Alternatives
While creatine monohydrate remains the gold standard, other forms have gained popularity, which is primarily due to good marketing

rather than scientific evidence. For example, creatine ethyl ester was initially promoted as a more bioavailable form, but studies revealed it to be less effective than monohydrate. Buffered creatine, marketed as Kre-Alkalyn, claims to reduce gastrointestinal discomfort, but there is little evidence to support this as a significant advantage. Creatine hydrochloride is water-soluble and may reduce bloating, but these effects are anecdotal, with no substantial research showing superiority over monohydrate.

Creatine and Cognitive Health
Beyond its physical benefits, creatine has garnered attention for its role in brain health. The brain relies heavily on ATP for energy, particularly during tasks requiring high cognitive effort. By replenishing brain phosphocreatine stores, creatine may improve mental performance, especially under conditions of sleep deprivation or stress. Studies in vegetarians, who typically have lower baseline creatine levels, show significant improvements in memory and cognitive function with supplementation. However, more research is needed in this area.

Doctor's Opinion: Creatine is a very common supplement and is perhaps one of the few truly useful supplements for performance enhancement. In addition, the literature has not shown any adverse effects with long term use. For doctors or anyone concerned about kidney health, it is important to highlight that creatine will not elevate creatinine levels. Patients who use creatine may have higher levels of muscle mass and therefore have higher baseline creatinine levels. This is why Cystatin C levels must be checked to accurately determine renal function.

Chapter 22: Androgenic Alopecia

Androgenic alopecia, commonly known as male-pattern baldness or female-pattern baldness, is the most prevalent form of hair loss in both men and women. It is a condition that affects millions globally and is characterized by a progressive thinning of hair that often results in noticeable bald patches or a significant reduction in hair density. This chapter will delve into the pathophysiology of androgenic alopecia, its genetic and hormonal underpinnings, diagnostic methods, treatment options, and the impact it has on those affected.

Pathophysiology and Genetics

Androgenic alopecia (male pattern baldness) is primarily influenced by genetic factors and hormonal imbalances. The condition is linked to the androgen hormone dihydrotestosterone (DHT), which is a derivative of testosterone. DHT forms from testosterone through the enzyme 5-alpha reductase. DHT is thought to bind to androgen receptors in the hair follicles, leading to a miniaturization of these follicles. This process results in progressively shorter and finer hair strands and, ultimately, a reduction in hair density.

At the molecular level, DHT alters the expression of various genes and proteins that regulate hair growth and follicle health. Once DHT binds to androgen receptors on hair follicle cells, it triggers downstream signaling that shortens the anagen (growth) phase of the hair cycle and prolongs the telogen (resting) phase. This cycle disruption reduces the time available for hair follicles to grow new, thick hair and increases the shedding of existing hairs. Additionally, DHT promotes increased expression of transforming growth factor-beta (TGF-β), which is known to induce apoptosis (cell death) in follicular keratinocytes, further impairing the ability of follicles to support healthy hair growth.

In AGA, follicular miniaturization is typically localized in specific scalp regions, such as the temples, crown, and frontal scalp, where androgen receptors are more densely expressed. This regional susceptibility is why hair loss in AGA follows a predictable pattern. The back and sides of the scalp, where hair follicles are less sensitive to DHT, are usually spared. Over time, affected follicles in susceptible areas undergo a progressive reduction in their size and function. The dermal papilla, a structure at the base of each follicle that provides nutrients and growth signals, becomes less effective, further limiting the follicle's ability to produce robust, terminal hairs.

Genetics play a significant role in androgenic alopecia. The condition follows a pattern of inheritance known as polygenic, which means that multiple genes contribute to its development. The most well-studied gene associated with androgenic alopecia is the AR gene, which encodes the androgen receptor. Variants of this gene can lead to increased sensitivity to androgens, thereby exacerbating the condition. Although the exact genetic pathways are complex and not entirely understood, having a family history of androgenic alopecia increases an individual's risk of developing the condition.

Hormonal Factors

Androgenic alopecia is not merely a result of aging but is significantly influenced by hormonal changes. Testosterone and DHT, its metabolite, play crucial roles in the development and progression of this type of hair loss. In men, DHT levels are higher and more influential, while in women, the balance of hormones such as estrogen and progesterone also affect hair growth and loss.

During puberty, an increase in androgen levels can trigger the onset of androgenic alopecia in genetically predisposed individuals. This also applies with the use of TRT, since more testosterone means more DHT and thereby the hair loss process is amplified. In women, changes in hormone levels, particularly during menopause, can also contribute to hair thinning. However, despite hormonal involvement, the exact mechanisms through which androgens lead to hair follicle miniaturization remain an area of active research.

Clinical Presentation and Diagnosis

Androgenic alopecia presents differently in men and women. In men, the condition typically begins with a receding hairline and thinning at the crown of the head. The pattern of hair loss often follows a distinctive M-shaped pattern, starting with the hairline retreating at the temples and thinning at the crown, eventually leading to a bald patch.

Diagnosis of androgenic alopecia is largely clinical, based on the pattern of hair loss and patient history. The patient's physician can generally make the likely diagnosis based on visual examination of the scalp. However, it is generally important to rule out any underlying causes such as hypothyroidism or iron deficiency. Sometimes autoimmune disease can also present with hair loss, such as lupus. In some cases, a scalp biopsy is necessary to make the diagnosis but not typically needed.

Treatment Options

Treatment for androgenic alopecia can be categorized into medical, surgical, and lifestyle interventions. The choice of treatment depends on the severity of hair loss, the patient's preferences, and their overall health.

Medical Treatments:

1. **Minoxidil:** Minoxidil is a topical treatment that is applied directly to the scalp. It is believed to work by increasing blood flow to hair follicles, thereby stimulating hair growth and slowing down hair loss. It is available over the counter in both 2% and 5% formulations though the 5% formulation is most commonly used. The 2% formulation was designed for use by women but, in practice, most women will use the 5% formulation. Minoxidil is effective in many but not all users, though, its exact mechanism of action is not fully understood. It is toxic to most household pets, especially cats, so pet owners should avoid the use of topical minoxidil.

Oral minoxidil is another option which generally leads to widespread hair growth and has been successfully used to treat various forms of alopecia including androgenic alopecia (male pattern baldness). Historically, it was a medication used to treat high blood pressure but is rarely used for that purpose nowadays. Most importantly, it carries a rare but very serious side effect of pericardial effusion (spontaneous development of fluid around the heart). This side effect is unrelated to the dosage and can happen at low doses. So, while it is a highly effective medication, and generally safe, it does carry a risk of a very serious side effect.

2. **Finasteride**: Finasteride is an oral medication that works by inhibiting the enzyme 5-alpha reductase, which converts testosterone into DHT. By reducing DHT levels, finasteride helps prevent further hair loss and can promote hair regrowth in some patients. It is very popular for treating male pattern baldness and has been used in combination with minoxidil. The popularity stems from the fact that it has been shown to be very effective. Dosages are generally 1mg daily, which is in contrast to 5mg daily doses used for treating benign prostate hyperplasia (BPH). For the vast majority of men, there are no side effects. However, there are uncommon side effects such as erectile dysfunction and libido changes.

The side effect potential of finasteride does deter some of its use. Post finasteride syndrome is one phrase that is commonly used on online platforms. The prevalence of side effects with finasteride use remains relatively low, in the single digit percentage range. While the risk does exist, it is quite uncommon. Those who are affected experience sexual dysfunction that is difficult to recover from. However, most users do not experience any side effects ever.

Another risk of finasteride is gynecomastia and male breast cancer. The true prevalence of gynecomastia is low amongst finasteride users and male breast cancer has been refuted in studies. For those who do not develop gynecomastia, breast cancer would be even more rare. As a starting point, male breast cancer is already rare to begin with. The evidence for this has been largely correlation and primarily seen in those using 5mg daily finasteride, as opposed to 1mg daily dosing which is what is used for male pattern baldness. However, it is a theoretical small risk that should be discussed between the patient and physician as part of informed decision making.

3. **Dutasteride**: Like finasteride, dutasteride is another oral medication that inhibits DHT production. It is sometimes used off-label for androgenic alopecia, particularly in cases where finasteride is not effective. However, its use is less common due to potential side effects and a less established track record for this specific indication. While it is very effective as it suppresses approximately 99% of serum DHT levels (in contrast to 70% for finasteride), the risk of adverse effects is naturally higher.

4. **Ketoconazole shampoo**: There is some evidence that ketoconazole shampoo, generally used to treat fungal related illness or dandruff, can aid in the treatment of male pattern baldness. Theoretically, it would lead to localized suppression of androgens. Its use would be typically 2-4 times per week. The evidence is generally weak, and, at best, it may be an adjunct agent. Sole use of this treatment is not recommended as it is unlikely to work, and it can cause excessively dry hair.

Surgical Treatments:

1. **Hair Transplant Surgery:** Hair transplant surgery involves relocating hair follicles from a donor site (usually the back or sides of the scalp) to the areas affected by hair loss. The two main techniques are follicular unit transplantation (FUT) and follicular unit extraction (FUE). FUT involves removing a strip of scalp tissue, while FUE involves extracting individual hair follicles. Both techniques can provide natural-looking results, but they require a skilled surgeon, a high price, and a recovery period.

Hair transplant surgery is generally the most proven procedural intervention for treating male pattern baldness.

2. **Scalp Reduction:** Scalp reduction surgery involves removing the bald areas of the scalp and stretching the remaining scalp to cover the area. This technique is less common today due to the associated risk of complications and the option of more advanced hair transplant methods.

3. **PRP:** Platelet-Rich Plasma (PRP) therapy is a treatment for hair loss that uses the patient's own blood to stimulate hair growth. PRP is derived by spinning a blood sample in a centrifuge to concentrate platelets, which are rich in growth factors that promote tissue repair and regeneration. When injected into the scalp, PRP enhances blood supply to hair follicles, prolongs the hair growth phase, and stimulates dormant follicles to produce thicker, healthier hair. It is commonly used to treat androgenetic alopecia (pattern hair loss) and other thinning conditions. Typically, patients undergo an initial series of three to four treatments spaced about four to six weeks apart, followed by maintenance sessions every 4-6 months to sustain results.

Lifestyle and Complementary Therapies:

1. **Nutritional Support**: While diet alone cannot cure or fix androgenic alopecia, maintaining a healthy diet rich in vitamins and minerals can support overall hair health and help maximize the benefit from any treatment modality. Nutrients such as biotin, iron, zinc, and omega-3 fatty acids are often recommended to help strengthen hair. However, none of these supplements in isolation will cure hair loss. In combination, they could have potential marginal benefits but, like most other supplements, their efficacy is mainly for individuals with nutrient deficiencies.

2. **Stress Management**: Chronic stress can exacerbate hair loss and can even cause severe hair loss called telogen effluvium. Techniques such as meditation, exercise, and counseling can help manage stress and potentially improve overall hair health.

3. **Cosmetic Solutions**: For those who do not wish to pursue medical or surgical treatments, cosmetic options such as hairpieces, wigs, and topical concealers can provide a temporary solution to hair loss.

Future Directions

Research into androgenic alopecia is ongoing, with several promising areas of investigation. Advances in genetics and molecular biology are providing deeper insights into the mechanisms of hair loss, potentially leading to more targeted and effective treatments. Stem cell research and regenerative medicine hold promise for developing new therapies that could reverse hair loss or regenerate hair follicles.

Additionally, new drugs and therapies are continually being tested, and ongoing clinical trials are exploring innovative treatments. The goal is to provide patients with more effective and personalized options to manage or even cure androgenic alopecia.

Conclusion

Androgenic alopecia is a complex condition with significant genetic and hormonal components. It affects millions of people worldwide and can have profound effects on an individual's appearance and self-esteem. While there are various treatment options available, each with its own benefits and limitations, ongoing research offers hope for more effective solutions in the future.

Understanding the pathophysiology, treatment options, and psychological impact of androgenic alopecia is essential for both patients and healthcare providers. By staying informed about the latest advancements and maintaining a comprehensive approach to treatment, individuals affected by androgenic alopecia can better manage their condition and improve their overall quality of life.

Chapter 23: Prostate Health: The Case for Screening

Prostate cancer is the second most common cancer among men worldwide and its impact is profound, affecting not only the individuals diagnosed but also their families and communities. The debate surrounding prostate cancer screening is intense, with arguments on both sides. However, this chapter will present a case in favor of prostate cancer screening, emphasizing the benefits it offers in terms of early detection, treatment, and overall patient outcomes.

Why is it relevant to this topic? The topics of TRT and PED use always have some degree of overlap with prostate health or at least raise questions and concerns about how they affect the prostate.

Prostate cancer screening has been controversial in medical circles for many years. The traditional approach was to screen all men in their 50s and older. This remained standard practice throughout the 2000s. However, newer studies and guidelines contradicted this practice, showing possible harm from universal screening. The idea was that slow-growing prostate cancer would not lead to mortality during the patient's natural life span and that treating it caused unnecessary harm. In the 2010s, many doctors switched to not universally screening and largely doing so for patients who requested it or had major risk factors. New literature showed an increase in metastatic prostate cancer and preventable morbidity and mortality. This was because many patients had faster growing prostate cancer or had much longer natural life expectancies. This led to the USPSTF modifying their guidelines. Some other nations also followed and lean towards recommending screening.

In the 2020s, we have better and more accurate screening modalities and many new treatment options. This increases accurate screening, while reducing side effects of treatment. The pendulum has swung back towards more screening based on newer evidence.

Testing Modalities

It is important to know that prostate cancer screening goes well beyond total PSA testing alone; it should be a multi-pronged approach that utilizes several testing strategies. There are different options that can be used depending on local resource availability and physician-patient shared decision making. These options include:

PHI (Prostate Health Index)
- Combines total PSA, free PSA, and [-2]proPSA (a PSA precursor) into a single score to assess prostate cancer risk.
- Offers improved specificity compared to PSA alone, reducing unnecessary biopsies.

4Kscore Test
- Measures four kallikrein proteins (total PSA, free PSA, intact PSA, and human kallikrein-2) and incorporates clinical information such as age and digital rectal exam results.
- Estimates the likelihood of finding high-grade prostate cancer on biopsy, helping guide decisions.

Understanding Prostate Cancer and Screening

Prostate cancer begins in the prostate, a small gland located below the bladder and in front of the rectum. It is a slow-growing cancer, but its progression can vary significantly. While some men with prostate cancer may live for years without symptoms or the need for treatment, others may experience aggressive forms of the disease that require immediate intervention. Screening aims to detect prostate cancer early, when it is most treatable and before it progresses to more advanced stages.

Early Detection and Improved Outcomes

One of the most compelling arguments in favor of prostate cancer screening is the potential for early detection. Early-stage prostate cancer often does not cause symptoms, making it difficult to detect without screening. When diagnosed early, the cancer is more likely to be confined to the prostate and less likely to have spread to other parts of the body.

Research has consistently shown that early detection can lead to better outcomes. The landmark Prostate, Lung, Colorectal, and Ovarian (PLCO) Cancer Screening Trial and the European Randomized Study of Screening for Prostate Cancer (ERSPC) are two major studies that have provided valuable insights into the benefits of screening. The ERSPC trial, for example, demonstrated that screening reduced prostate cancer mortality by approximately 20%. This reduction is significant, especially considering the impact of early diagnosis on survival rates.

Early detection through screening allows for a range of treatment options, from less invasive approaches like active surveillance to more aggressive treatments if necessary. For many men, early intervention can mean the difference between a manageable disease and one that requires more intensive and potentially life-altering treatments.

Reducing Mortality and Improving Quality of Life
The primary goal of prostate cancer screening is to reduce mortality rates. The evidence supporting this objective is robust. The reduction in prostate cancer deaths as a result of screening is a key factor in favor of this approach. Men who undergo regular screening have a better chance of discovering the disease before it progresses to a more advanced stage, thereby improving their chances of survival. The most up-to-date studies support this point, while the old literature opposed screening.

Additionally, the quality of life for men diagnosed with prostate cancer at an early stage is often better than for those diagnosed later. Early-stage cancer treatment typically involves less aggressive therapies and can be managed with fewer side effects. For instance, many men with early prostate cancer may be candidates for active surveillance, which involves monitoring the cancer closely rather than undergoing immediate treatment. This approach can help avoid unnecessary side effects and maintain a higher quality of life.

Addressing Concerns and Mitigating Risks
While the benefits of screening are significant, it is also important to address concerns associated with prostate cancer screening, such as overdiagnosis and overtreatment. Overdiagnosis occurs when screening detects cancers that would not have caused harm during the patient's lifetime. This can lead to overtreatment, where patients undergo treatments that may not be necessary, potentially causing more harm than benefit.

However, advancements in screening technology and improved risk stratification methods have helped address these concerns. Modern screening approaches use a combination of PSA levels, genetic markers, and imaging techniques to better identify which cancers are likely to be aggressive and which are not. For example, the use of multiparametric MRI (mpMRI) has enhanced the ability to detect clinically significant cancers while reducing the likelihood of detecting indolent forms of the disease. The risk of prostate biopsy is also relatively low, contrary to the more traditional thinking of the 2010s.

Moreover, shared decision-making between patients and healthcare providers is crucial. By discussing the potential benefits and risks of screening, patients can make informed choices about their care. This personalized approach helps ensure that screening decisions align with the individual's health goals and values.

The Role of Screening in Special Populations
Screening is particularly important for certain populations at higher risk for prostate cancer. Men with a family history of prostate cancer or those of African descent are at an increased risk and may benefit more from early screening. The American Urological Association and other professional organizations recommend earlier and more frequent screening for these high-risk groups.

Family history plays a significant role in prostate cancer risk. Men with a first-degree relative (father or brother) who had prostate cancer are at a higher risk of developing the disease themselves. For these individuals, early screening can be especially beneficial in catching the disease at a manageable stage.

Similarly, African American men are statistically more likely to develop prostate cancer and to do so at a younger age. For these men, the potential benefits of early detection through screening may outweigh the risks, making a strong case for regular screening.

The Economic Perspective
Economic considerations also play a role in the debate over prostate cancer screening. While screening involves costs, the long-term benefits often outweigh these initial expenses. Early detection and treatment of prostate cancer can reduce the need for more extensive and costly interventions later on. Furthermore, the reduction in mortality and improvement in quality of life for patients who are diagnosed early can lead to overall cost savings in the healthcare system.

Preventive measures, such as screening, can be viewed as an investment in health that yields returns in terms of reduced treatment costs and improved patient outcomes. By discovering prostate cancer early, healthcare systems can potentially avoid the higher costs associated with advanced disease management and palliative care.

Conclusion
The case for prostate cancer screening is compelling when using the most up to date literature. The ability to detect prostate cancer early, when it is most treatable and before it progresses to advanced stages, offers significant obvious benefits. Early detection improves survival rates, enhances the quality of life for patients, and can be particularly valuable for high-risk populations.

While concerns about overdiagnosis and overtreatment exist, advancements in screening technology and personalized approaches have addressed many of these issues. Shared decision-making between patients and healthcare providers ensures that screening decisions are tailored to individual needs and preferences.

Ultimately, prostate cancer screening represents a crucial tool in the fight against one of the most common cancers affecting men today. The benefits of early detection, improved treatment options, and reduced mortality rates make a strong case for screening, affirming its role as a vital component of proactive healthcare for men.

Chapter 24: Comprehensive Overview of Cardiac Health and Lipid Management

Introduction

Cardiac health is a critical aspect of overall well-being, with cardiovascular disease (CVD) being a leading cause of morbidity and mortality worldwide. The management of cardiac health encompasses understanding and addressing risk factors such as high cholesterol and lipid disorders. This chapter provides an in-depth exploration of these factors, including various lipid tests, treatments, lifestyle modifications, as well as advanced diagnostic tools such as coronary calcium scores and stress tests.

Atherosclerosis and Coronary Artery Disease

Atherosclerosis is a chronic, progressive disease characterized by the accumulation of plaque in the walls of arteries. It begins with endothelial dysfunction, where damage to the inner lining of arteries occurs due to factors such as hypertension, smoking, high cholesterol, or inflammation. In response to this injury, low-density lipoprotein (LDL) cholesterol particles infiltrate the damaged area and become oxidized. This triggers an immune response, where macrophages engulf the oxidized LDL, forming foam cells, and initiating the development of a fatty streak. Over time, smooth muscle cells migrate to the area and produce a fibrous cap over the fatty deposit, forming a plaque.

As the plaque grows, it narrows the artery, reducing blood flow and increasing the risk of rupture. If the plaque ruptures, it exposes the underlying materials, leading to the formation of a blood clot (thrombus) that can further obstruct blood flow. This process plays a critical role in the development of coronary artery disease (CAD), where the coronary arteries that supply blood to the heart become narrowed or blocked. Reduced blood flow to the heart muscle can result in chest pain (angina) or, if the blood flow is severely restricted or blocked completely, a myocardial infarction (heart attack) occurs.

Risk factors for the development of atherosclerosis and CAD include high LDL cholesterol, low high-density lipoprotein (HDL) cholesterol, hypertension, smoking, diabetes, obesity, and a sedentary lifestyle. Management involves reducing these risk factors through lifestyle modifications, medications to lower cholesterol and blood pressure, and, in some cases, surgical interventions like angioplasty or coronary artery bypass grafting (CABG) to restore blood flow.

Stroke

A stroke occurs when the blood supply to part of the brain is interrupted or reduced, depriving brain tissue of oxygen and nutrients. This can happen due to the blockage of an artery (ischemic stroke) or the rupture of a blood vessel (hemorrhagic stroke). In an ischemic stroke, atherosclerosis can contribute to the formation of a blood clot that obstructs blood flow in a cerebral artery.

Understanding Cholesterol and Lipid Disorders

The Basics of Cholesterol and Lipids

Cholesterol and lipids are essential for various bodily functions, including cell membrane structure and hormone production. However, imbalances in these substances can lead to cardiovascular disease. Cholesterol is carried in the blood by lipoproteins; understanding the different types of lipoproteins and their implications is crucial for effective management.

- **Low-Density Lipoprotein (LDL):** Often referred to as "bad" cholesterol, LDL carries cholesterol from the liver to the cells. High levels of LDL can lead to plaque buildup in the arteries, increasing the risk of heart disease.
- **High-Density Lipoprotein (HDL):** Known as "good" cholesterol, HDL helps remove excess cholesterol from the bloodstream and transport it back to the liver for excretion. Higher levels of HDL are associated with a lower risk of heart disease. There are subtypes of HDL, but with little clinical relevance.

- **Total Cholesterol:** This is the sum of LDL, HDL, and other lipid components in the blood. While useful, it is less informative than the breakdown of different types of lipoproteins.
- **Apolipoprotein B100 (ApoB100):** ApoB100 is a protein found on LDL particles as well as IDL (intermediate density cholesterol), VLDL (very low-density cholesterol) and lipoprotein (a). It is considered a better indicator of cardiovascular risk than LDL alone.
- **Lipoprotein(a) [Lp(a)]:** Lp(a) is a type of lipoprotein that carries cholesterol and is genetically determined. Elevated levels of Lp(a) are associated with an increased risk of cardiovascular disease, independent of other lipid measures.
- **Triglycerides:** Triglycerides are a type of fat (lipid) found in your blood, formed from the calories you consumed but did not use immediately. Excess triglycerides are then stored in fat cells for energy. High triglyceride levels are an indicator of metabolic disease.
- **Very Low-Density Lipoprotein (VLDL):** VLDL is a type of lipoprotein responsible for transporting triglycerides from the liver to peripheral tissues for energy or storage. Like LDL, it is considered atherogenic, as high levels can contribute to plaque formation in arterial walls. VLDL is rich in triglycerides, and as it delivers these fats, it is metabolized into intermediate-density lipoprotein (IDL), a precursor to LDL. Elevated VLDL levels are often associated with metabolic disorders, such as insulin resistance and type 2 diabetes, and are considered a marker of increased cardiovascular risk. However, it is not routinely measured as it rarely alters management.
- **Intermediate-Density Lipoprotein (IDL):** IDL represents a transitional lipoprotein formed as VLDL sheds triglycerides and is remodeled in the bloodstream. It carries both cholesterol and triglycerides but is less triglyceride-rich than VLDL. IDL can either be taken up by the liver for clearance or further metabolized into LDL. Persistently high levels of IDL are associated with atherogenesis and are indicative of an impaired

lipid metabolism. Although less commonly measured in clinical practice, elevated IDL is another factor contributing to cardiovascular disease risk.

Lipid Testing and Interpretation

Common Lipid Tests
- **Lipid Panel:** A lipid panel measures total cholesterol, LDL, HDL, and triglycerides. This test is fundamental in assessing lipid levels and guiding treatment.
- **Apolipoprotein B100:** This test quantifies the number of LDL particles and can provide a more accurate assessment of cardiovascular risk than LDL cholesterol alone. This is particularly useful for those with high triglyceride levels as determining the LDL level is not possible.
- **Lipoprotein(a):** Measured through a specific blood test, elevated Lp(a) levels can indicate a higher risk of cardiovascular events, particularly if other risk factors are present. It is recommended to test Lp(a) once in everyone's lifetime.

Interpretation of Results
- **LDL (Low-Density Lipoprotein):**
  - Optimal: <100 mg/dL (<2.6 mmol/L)
  - Near optimal: 100-129 mg/dL (2.6–3.3 mmol/L)
  - Borderline high: 130-159 mg/dL (3.4–4.1 mmol/L)
  - High: 160-189 mg/dL (4.1–4.9 mmol/L)
  - Very high: ≥190 mg/dL (≥4.9 mmol/L)
- **HDL (High-Density Lipoprotein):**
  - High (protective): >60 mg/dL (>1.55 mmol/L)
  - Low (risk factor): <40 mg/dL (<1.03 mmol/L)
- **Total Cholesterol:**
  - Desirable: <200 mg/dL (<5.2 mmol/L)
  - Borderline high: 200-239 mg/dL (5.2–6.2 mmol/L)
  - High: ≥240 mg/dL (≥6.2 mmol/L)

- **ApoB100 (Apolipoprotein B):**

- o Varies by lab, but generally <90 mg/dL (<0.9 g/L) is considered optimal.
- **Lipoprotein(a):**
  - o Optimal levels: <30 mg/dL (<75 nmol/L)
  - o Higher levels are associated with increased risk

Novel Lipid Tests:
- **LDL Particle Number (LDL-P):** Measures the number of LDL particles, which may better reflect cardiovascular risk than LDL cholesterol levels alone. Although, this is only theoretical.
- **LDL Particle Size:** Evaluates the size of LDL particles since small, dense LDL particles are more atherogenic (likely to cause plaques) than large, buoyant ones. Again, this is only theoretical.
- **Remnant Cholesterol:** Represents cholesterol carried in triglyceride-rich lipoproteins (VLDL and IDL); high levels are linked to residual cardiovascular risk, though, measuring this is largely academic.
- **Apolipoprotein A-I (ApoA-I):** Major protein in HDL particles; low levels may indicate reduced reverse cholesterol transport capacity. It is effectively a surrogate marker for HDL but can be used in a ratio with ApoB levels to guide lipid risk factors.
- **Apolipoprotein C-III (ApoC-III):** Involved in triglyceride metabolism; elevated levels are associated with increased cardiovascular risk and hypertriglyceridemia.
- **Non-HDL Cholesterol:** Total cholesterol minus HDL cholesterol, representing all atherogenic particles, including LDL, VLDL, and remnants.
- **Oxidized LDL (OxLDL):** Measures LDL particles modified by oxidation; higher levels are associated with increased plaque formation and cardiovascular risk. Although, there is not much clinical data to show utility in checking this.
- **Lipoprotein-associated Phospholipase A2 (Lp-PLA2):** An enzyme linked to vascular inflammation and plaque instability; high levels indicate a higher risk of atherosclerosis and cardiovascular events.

- **Chylomicron Remnants:** Measures postprandial lipoproteins involved in fat transport; elevated levels are linked to atherogenesis.

Treatment Strategies for Dyslipidemia

1. **Lifestyle and Dietary Modifications**

Dietary Changes
- **Reducing Saturated and Trans Fats:** Saturated fats (found in red meat, butter, etc.) and trans fats (found in many processed foods) can raise LDL cholesterol levels. Reducing these fats can improve lipid profiles. The reduction should be gradual as people often report changes in energy levels when experiencing a sudden reduction in saturated fat and trans fat intake.
- **Increasing Fibre Intake:** Soluble fibre (found in oats, beans, apples, etc.) aids in reducing LDL cholesterol by binding bile acids and promoting their excretion. A steady and gradual increase in fibre intake leads to a significant improvement in the lipid profile.
- **Incorporating Healthy Fats:** Monounsaturated and polyunsaturated fats (found in olive oil, avocados, nuts, etc.) can help lower LDL cholesterol and improve overall lipid profiles.
- **Omega-3 Fatty Acids:** Omega-3 fatty acids (found in fish, chia seeds, flax seeds, etc.) have been shown to lower triglycerides and have anti-inflammatory effects. However, studies have shown mixed efficacy and long-term risks. Vascepa, which is a high dose EPA (an omega 3 fatty acid), has been shown to have clinical benefit in certain heart disease patients. The DHA component in omega 3s could pose an increased risk of atrial fibrillation and the cardiac benefit generally seems to be limited to EPA only.

Lifestyle Changes

- **Regular Exercise:** Physical activity helps increase HDL cholesterol, lower LDL cholesterol, and lower triglycerides. Individuals hoping to improve their lipid profiles with the help of regular exercise should aim for at least 150 minutes of moderate-intensity exercise per week.
- **Weight Management:** Maintaining a healthy weight can help improve lipid levels and reduce the risk of heart disease.
- **Smoking Cessation:** Smoking is a major risk factor for cardiovascular disease, and it can lower HDL cholesterol. Quitting smoking can improve heart health and lipid levels.
- **Moderate Alcohol Consumption:** Excessive alcohol can raise triglyceride levels. Moderate consumption, if any, is recommended for heart health.

2. Pharmacological Treatments

- **Statins:** Statins are the first-line treatment for high LDL cholesterol. They work by inhibiting HMG-CoA reductase, an enzyme involved in cholesterol production. Common statins include atorvastatin, simvastatin, and rosuvastatin. Statins which are hydrophilic, such as rosuvastatin, are less likely to induce side effects like muscle pains.
- **Ezetimibe:** Ezetimibe works by blocking the absorption of cholesterol in the intestine, which helps lower LDL levels. It is often used in combination with statins when additional LDL reduction is needed. Monotherapy with ezetimibe is not usually recommended, other than rare conditions such as sitosterolemia
- **Bempedoic Acid:** Bempedoic acid is a newer medication that inhibits ATP citrate lyase, an enzyme involved in cholesterol synthesis. It is used for patients who cannot tolerate statins or need additional LDL lowering.
- **PCSK9 Inhibitors:** PCSK9 inhibitors, such as evolocumab and alirocumab, are potent monoclonal antibodies that help lower LDL cholesterol by increasing the liver's ability to remove LDL from the blood. They are typically used in patients with familia

hypercholesterolemia or those who require significant LDL reduction.
- **Niacin:** Niacin was historically used to treat high cholesterol levels, specifically LDL. It was newly found to decrease lipoprotein (a) levels as well. It usually would lead to flushing sensations as a side effect. However, niacin also raised homocysteine levels which is another known 'bad" biological marker in the context of coronary artery disease risk development. The issue with niacin has been that despite lowering certain pathogenic markers, it has not been shown in studies to decrease the risk of heart disease. Hence, cardiology associations do not recommend its use. It also carries the risk of liver toxicity, though, this tends to be inconsistent.
- **Vascepa:** Vascepa consists of high-dose omega-3 fatty acids, specifically eicosapentaenoic acid (EPA). It is recommended only for individuals with elevated triglyceride levels and existing heart disease. Like all omega-3s, it is intended for those with very high triglyceride levels. Omega-3s are not generally recommended for routine use, particularly for preventing heart disease. While omega-3 supplements can mildly raise LDL levels, this effect is mostly seen with docosahexaenoic acid (DHA), not EPA, which is the active ingredient in Vascepa.
- **Cholestyramine:** A bile acid binding drug that is usually used to treat subtypes of chronic diarrhea, it was also used to treat cholesterol. Given the development of newer drugs, it has fallen out of favor. It is however considered safe in pregnancy and has remained one of the very few theoretical options for treating very severe cholesterol disorders while pregnant.
- **Inclirisan:** A newer agent that has similar potency to PSK9 inhibitors in treating severely elevated cholesterol.
- **Febofibrate (and other Fibrates):** Primarily a drug used to treat severely high triglycerides with only modest benefit on other lipid markers. It does have potential gastrointestinal adverse effects.

3. Supplements for Cholesterol Management
- **Plant Sterols and Stanols**
  - **Benefit:** Block cholesterol absorption in the intestine, potentially lowering LDL cholesterol by 6-15%.
  - **Risk:** Can cause digestive issues such as bloating and diarrhea. They do not significantly impact overall cardiovascular outcomes, so their benefit in routine use is unclear. One key point to highlight is that a lot of medications and supplements can alter a biomarker on lab tests without changing the outcome of disease prevention.
- **Red Yeast Rice**
  - **Benefit:** Contains monacolin K, which mimics low-dose statins in lowering LDL cholesterol.
  - **Risk:** Can cause similar side effects to statins, such as muscle pain and liver toxicity. Quality control issues with supplements are common, with some containing unsafe contaminants. Logically, since they are very similar, it makes more sense to take a statin instead.
- **Soluble Fibre (e.g., Psyllium)**
  - **Benefit:** Reduces LDL cholesterol modestly by binding to cholesterol in the gut.
  - **Risk:** Can cause bloating, gas, and reduced absorption of certain medications, if not taken properly. Although, this is generally when consuming higher doses.
- **Garlic Extract**
  - **Benefit:** Some studies suggest it may lower LDL cholesterol slightly, though the effects are minimal and inconsistent.
  - **Risk:** Can cause bad breath, gastrointestinal discomfort, and bleeding risk when combined with anticoagulants.
- **Coenzyme Q10 (CoQ10)**
  - **Benefit:** Commonly used to reduce statin-related muscle pain, though, evidence is mixed.
  - **Risk:** Offers no direct cholesterol-lowering benefit and may interact with certain medications. The theoretical mechanism was promising but studies failed to show any

benefit. Although, anecdotal evidence supporting the use of coenzyme Q10 remains quite strong.
- **Policosanol**
  - **Benefit:** Initially thought to lower LDL cholesterol and raise HDL, but evidence supporting its efficacy is weak and largely based on non-independent studies.
  - **Risk:** Side effects include headaches and gastrointestinal upset. Overall, its utility is questionable.
- **Artichoke Leaf Extract**
  - **Benefit:** May slightly lower total cholesterol by improving bile flow.
  - **Risk:** Effectiveness is limited, and it can cause digestive side effects or allergic reactions in individuals sensitive to plants like ragweed.
- **Bergamot Extract**
  - **Benefit:** Contains flavonoids that may modestly lower LDL cholesterol and triglycerides.
  - **Risk:** Long-term safety data is lacking, and it may not provide consistent results across different populations.
- **Green Tea Extract**
  - **Benefit:** Rich in catechins, which may lower LDL cholesterol marginally when consumed in large amounts.
  - **Risk:** High doses can lead to liver toxicity, gastrointestinal upset, and caffeine-related side effects like jitteriness.

Special considerations for athletes, bodybuilders and recreational lifters with elevated cholesterol

High cholesterol can exist in many athletes and active individuals who consume very healthy diets. Often, it is due to genetics, especially high LDL cholesterol. In fact, in middle aged athletes, the most common cause of heart disease is coronary artery disease caused by genetic risk factors including high cholesterol. For those who have abnormal cholesterol despite extensive exercise and a healthy optimized diet, pharmacologic intervention is often necessary. Of course, as mentioned previously in this book, those on anabolic steroid may suffer from abnormal cholesterol as a direct result of their PED use. This can be reversed by discontinuation or minimization of use. However, if the decision is made to start medication, the question is which one?

This is often an important consideration as many cholesterol medications carry an adverse effect of muscle through aches, pains, and even, potentially, muscle breakdown. This is usually not a major concern for the average person, as these adverse effects are not as noticeable. However, it can be a major concern for a high-performance athlete or even recreational lifters. Statins for example, could potentially hinder peak performance despite being a great drug for dyslipidemia. For those with confirmed coronary artery disease, statin therapy is necessary. However, for those without coronary artery disease who only require LDL reduction, a discussion about medication selection is encouraged.

Most lipid medications will not cause side effects, most of the time. However, they could have marginal effects on performance, especially peak muscle growth and strength. Hydrophilic statins, like rosuvastatin, are less likely to cause muscle related side effects and would be a preferred option. Depending on the context, lab findings, and athletic goals, a low dose or a reduction in dose frequency may be an option. Another option could be monotherapy with ezetimibe, if the individual wants to strictly avoid statins. While not as effective as statins, some reduction in LDL with the use of ezetimibe is better than none. PCKS9 inhibitors are also an excellent option for those with very high LDL levels who may require high intensity statins (potentially combination therapy with other oral medications) and would be less likely to hinder athletic performance. However, cost ma be a limitation.

Other medications that would not be recommended are fibrates, niacin bile acid binders, and bempedoic acid. Fibrates have a larger adverse effect potential while niacin has not been shown to be effective in hea disease prevention. At this stage, bempedoic acid is premature and may present risks to athletes, especially with monotherapy.

Coenzyme Q10 and Use in Athletes

Coenzyme Q10 (CoQ10) is a fat-soluble compound found in mitochondria, where it plays a critical role in energy production and serves as a powerful antioxidant. Statins, which inhibit cholesterol synthesis, can also reduce CoQ10 levels since the biosynthesis pathways of both molecules overlap. This depletion is often hypothesized to contribute to statin-associated muscle symptoms (SAMS), such as pain or weakness. While CoQ10 supplementation has been studied for alleviating these symptoms, results are mixed. Some randomized controlled trials suggest modest reductions in muscle pain, while others show no significant benefit compared to placebo. Anecdotally, some patients report relief of muscle symptoms with CoQ10 use, though this may be influenced by the placebo effect. Despite its safety profile, evidence does not consistently support CoQ10 as a universal remedy for SAMS, and its routine use in conjunction with statins is not broadly recommended.

However, its use in high-performance athletes who also use statins has not been studied. It is more likely to be useful in athletes simply because the threshold for benefit is vastly different than the general population. Elite athletes are very often looking for any marginal or even miniscule benefit. If statins were to lead to even the slightest performance deficit, that would have a major impact on competition outcomes. Now if this deficit can be offset by coenzyme q10 use, then the benefit is substantial even if the magnitude is quite low for the general population. Since this has not been studied adequately, no conclusions can be made at this time.

Advanced Cardiac Diagnostic Tools

Coronary Calcium Score

The coronary calcium score is a measure of the amount of calcium in the coronary arteries, which is indicative of atherosclerotic plaque. A higher score suggests a greater degree of coronary artery disease (CAD) and can help stratify risk, particularly in asymptomatic individuals. In layman's terms, patients who never experience any chest pain can see if they have any evidence of underlying coronary artery disease.

Scoring:
- **0**: No identifiable coronary artery disease
- **1-100**: Mild coronary artery disease
- **101-400**: Moderate coronary artery disease
- **>400**: Severe coronary artery disease

Coronary CT Angiography (CTA)
Coronary CT angiography provides detailed images of the coronary arteries and is used to evaluate the presence and extent of coronary artery disease. It can identify blockages and is useful in assessing patients with intermediate risk or those who cannot undergo invasive coronary angiography.

Benefits:
- Non-invasive
- Provides detailed 3D images
- Helps in planning treatment strategies
- 99% specific for coronary artery disease; a negative or normal test rules out coronary artery disease

For Doctors: Keep in mind that coronary calcium score testing and coronary CT scans are not the exact same test. Coronary CTs include calcium score testing, but ordering a coronary calcium score only will not provide the anatomical details of a coronary CT. The coronary CT scan specifically outlines the anatomy and presence of any plaque buildup.

Homocysteine – What's the deal?
Homocysteine is an amino acid derived from methionine metabolism which plays a role in various biochemical pathways, including methylation and sulfur transfer. Elevated levels of homocysteine, known as hyperhomocysteinemia, have been associated with an increased risk of cardiovascular diseases, such as atherosclerosis, stroke, and venous thromboembolism. The proposed mechanism

involves endothelial damage, oxidative stress, and enhanced clot formation, all of which can contribute to vascular injury. Homocysteine levels are influenced by genetic factors, such as MTHFR mutations, as well as deficiencies in vitamins B6, B12, and folate, which are critical for its metabolism.

Evidence and Screening
While early studies suggested a strong link between elevated homocysteine and cardiovascular disease, more recent research has questioned its role as a direct cause. Large-scale randomized controlled trials have shown that lowering homocysteine levels through supplementation with B vitamins does not significantly reduce cardiovascular events. As a result, most cardiology societies, including the American Heart Association (AHA), do not recommend routine screening for homocysteine levels in the general population. Testing may be reserved for specific cases, such as individuals with early-onset cardiovascular disease or a history of unexplained thromboembolism, where a hereditary or metabolic cause is suspected. It is also used in the workup of certain vitamin deficiencies. Ultimately, if lowering it did play a role in preventing heart disease, then the use of B12 supplements would lower heart disease in the general population. However, it does not.

Treatment and Implications
In theory, elevated homocysteine levels can be treated with supplementation of folate, vitamin B6, and vitamin B12, which are cofactors in its metabolism. This approach can effectively lower homocysteine levels but has not been proven to translate into meaningful reductions in cardiovascular risk. The broader implications of homocysteine extend beyond heart disease, as elevated levels have also been associated with cognitive decline, osteoporosis, and pregnancy complications. While homocysteine remains a marker of interest, current guidelines emphasize addressing traditional risk factors, such as lipid levels, hypertension, and lifestyle habits, over targeting homocysteine specifically. It serves as a reminder that complex metabolic markers must be interpreted within the context of

overall cardiovascular risk. And that isolating markers on their own may not be useful.

Stress Tests and Other Heart Disease Screenings
Types of Stress Tests
- **Exercise Stress Test:** This test involves walking on a treadmill or pedaling a stationary bike while monitoring heart rate, blood pressure, and ECG. It helps assess how well the heart copes with physical stress. It is a commonly used stress test modality around the world but does come with major limitations in truly determining the existence of heart disease.
- **Pharmacologic Stress Test:** For patients unable to exercise, medications are used to stimulate the heart as if it were under stress. This is often combined with imaging techniques like echocardiography or nuclear imaging. Nuclear imaging is a highly accurate modality of stress testing and is the preferred stress test modality.
- **Stress Echocardiogram:** This involves an ultrasound of the heart during stress to evaluate cardiac function and detect areas of poor blood flow.
- **Nuclear Stress Test:** Radioactive tracers are used to visualize blood flow to the heart muscle during stress, helping to identify areas with reduced blood flow. This is the most accurate modality of stress testing.

Other Diagnostic Tests
- **Electrocardiogram (ECG):** An ECG records the electrical activity of the heart and can detect arrhythmias, previous heart attacks, and other heart conditions. While it is a very simple and quick test, it remains controversial on whether to obtain it on someone without any symptoms.
- **Holter Monitor:** This portable device records the heart's electrical activity over 24-48 hours and is useful for detecting intermittent arrhythmias. This is generally intended for patients who have symptoms only, such as palpations.

Conclusion

Maintaining cardiac health is a multifaceted process that involves understanding and managing lipid levels, adopting lifestyle changes, and utilizing advanced diagnostic tools. High cholesterol and lipid disorders are critical risk factors for cardiovascular disease. Effective management of these conditions includes both pharmacological treatments and lifestyle modifications. Regular screening and appropriate use of diagnostic tests, such as coronary calcium scores and stress tests, play a vital role in early detection and management of heart disease.

For individuals with high cholesterol or other risk factors, collaborating with one's doctor to develop a personalized plan is essential. This plan should integrate medical treatments, dietary and lifestyle changes, and regular monitoring to optimize heart health and reduce the risk of cardiovascular events.

Chapter 25: Metabolic Syndrome: Understanding the Epidemic of Modern Times

Introduction

Metabolic syndrome is an increasingly prevalent health condition characterized by a cluster of metabolic disorders that heighten an individual's risk of developing cardiovascular disease, type 2 diabetes, and other serious health issues. This syndrome reflects a complex interplay of genetic, environmental, and lifestyle factors, making it a significant concern in public health.

Defining Metabolic Syndrome

Metabolic syndrome is defined by a combination of conditions that occur together, increasing the risk of heart disease, stroke, and type 2 diabetes. According to the National Heart, Lung, and Blood Institute (NHLBI), the syndrome is characterized by three or more of the following criteria:

- **Abdominal Obesity**: Measured by waist circumference, where men with a waist circumference of 40 inches or more and women with 35 inches or more are considered at risk.
- **Hyperglycemia**: Elevated fasting blood glucose levels of 100 mg/dL or higher, or a diagnosis of type 2 diabetes.
- **Hypertension**: Elevated blood pressure, typically defined as 130/85 mm Hg or higher.
- **Dyslipidemia**: Abnormal lipid levels, specifically high levels of triglycerides (150 mg/dL or more) and/or low levels of high-density lipoprotein (HDL) cholesterol (less than 40 mg/dL in men and less than 50 mg/dL in women).
- **Insulin Resistance**: Often measured indirectly by elevated blood glucose levels or through other markers such as fasting insulin levels.

Causes and Risk Factors

Metabolic syndrome is the result of a combination of genetic predispositions and lifestyle factors. Here's a closer look at the primary contributors:

- **Genetic Factors**: Certain genetic traits increase susceptibility to metabolic syndrome. Variations in genes related to insulin signaling, lipid metabolism, and fat storage can predispose individuals to the syndrome. However, genetics alone are not determinative; environmental and lifestyle factors play a significant role.
- **Obesity**: Central obesity, or excess fat around the abdomen, is a significant risk factor for metabolic syndrome. Adipose tissue, especially visceral fat, secretes hormones and cytokines that can lead to inflammation, insulin resistance, and other metabolic disturbances.
- **Physical Inactivity**: Sedentary behavior contributes to obesity and metabolic dysfunction. Regular physical activity helps regulate blood glucose levels, reduce blood pressure, and improve lipid profiles, thereby mitigating the risk of metabolic syndrome.
- **Unhealthy Diet**: Diets high in refined carbohydrates, sugars, and unhealthy fats contribute to weight gain and metabolic abnormalities. Conversely, diets rich in whole grains, fruits, vegetables, and healthy fats are protective against metabolic syndrome.
- **Insulin Resistance**: Insulin resistance, where cells do not respond effectively to insulin, is a core component of metabolic syndrome. This condition leads to higher blood glucose levels and increased insulin production, which can eventually result in type 2 diabetes.
- **Genetics and Ethnicity**: Certain ethnic groups, such as individuals of South Asian or Hispanic descent, are at higher risk for developing metabolic syndrome. These groups often experience higher rates of central obesity and insulin resistance.
- **Age and Gender**: Metabolic syndrome prevalence increases with age, and postmenopausal women are at a higher risk due to hormonal changes that affect fat distribution and metabolism.

Health Implications
The consequences of metabolic syndrome are far-reaching and potentially severe. These consequences include:
- **Cardiovascular Disease**: Individuals with metabolic syndrome have a significantly higher risk of developing heart disease. The combination of hypertension, dyslipidemia, and obesity contributes to atherosclerosis, which can lead to heart attacks and strokes.
- **Type 2 Diabetes**: Insulin resistance, a hallmark of metabolic syndrome, is closely linked to the development of type 2 diabetes. Persistent high blood glucose levels can lead to complications such as neuropathy, nephropathy, and retinopathy
- **Fatty Liver Disease**: Non-alcoholic fatty liver disease (NAFLD) is common among individuals with metabolic syndrome. Excessive fat accumulation in the liver can lead to inflammation, fibrosis, and eventually cirrhosis.
- **Polycystic Ovary Syndrome (PCOS)**: Women with metabolic syndrome are at higher risk for PCOS, a condition characterized by irregular menstrual cycles, infertility, and excessive androgen levels.
- **Sleep Apnea**: Obesity and metabolic syndrome are associated with obstructive sleep apnea, a condition where the airway becomes blocked during sleep, leading to fragmented sleep and increased cardiovascular risk.

Diagnosis and Screening
Diagnosing metabolic syndrome involves assessing the presence of multiple risk factors. A thorough evaluation includes:
- **Medical History and Physical Examination**: Assessing symptoms, lifestyle factors, and family history can provide insight into the likelihood of metabolic syndrome. A significant caloric surplus and intake of large amounts of ultra-processed food is a major risk factor.

- **Laboratory Tests**: Blood tests are used to measure fasting glucose levels, lipid profiles, and other biomarkers that indicate metabolic disturbances.
- **Body Measurements**: Waist circumference and body mass index (BMI) measurements help assess obesity and fat distribution.
- **Blood Pressure Monitoring**: Regular monitoring of blood pressure is essential for detecting hypertension, a key component of metabolic syndrome.

Management and Prevention

Managing and preventing metabolic syndrome involves a multifaceted approach:
- **Lifestyle Modifications**: Adopting a healthy lifestyle is the cornerstone of managing metabolic syndrome. This includes:
  - **Diet**: Emphasizing a balanced diet rich in fruits, vegetables, whole grains, lean proteins, and healthy fats. Reducing intake of processed foods, sugary beverages, and trans fats is crucial.
  - **Exercise**: Engaging in regular physical activity, such as brisk walking, cycling, or swimming, can help reduce weight, improve insulin sensitivity, and lower blood pressure.
  - **Weight Management**: Achieving and maintaining a healthy weight through diet and exercise is critical for managing metabolic syndrome. Even modest weight loss can lead to significant improvements in metabolic health.
- **Medical Interventions**: In some cases, medication may be necessary to address specific components of metabolic syndrome. These medications include:
  - **Antihypertensives**: The DASH diet is quite useful for lowering blood pressure. If the blood pressure is too high or lifestyle changes are unsuccessful, then medications to control high blood pressure can be started.

- o **Statins**: To manage dyslipidemia and reduce cholesterol levels.
- o **Metformin**: Commonly prescribed for insulin resistance and type 2 diabetes.
- **Regular Monitoring**: Ongoing monitoring of blood glucose levels, blood pressure, and lipid profiles is essential for tracking progress and adjusting treatment as needed.
- **Education and Support**: Providing education on healthy lifestyle choices and access to support resources, such as counseling or weight loss programs, can enhance adherence to lifestyle changes and improve outcomes.

Conclusion

Metabolic syndrome represents a complex and growing health challenge in the modern world. It reflects the intersection of genetics, lifestyle, and environmental factors, manifesting as a cluster of conditions that significantly increase the risk of serious diseases. Effective management and prevention require a comprehensive approach that includes lifestyle modifications, medical interventions, and ongoing monitoring. By addressing the underlying causes and promoting healthier habits, individuals can reduce their risk and improve their overall well-being. Public health initiatives and personal health strategies must work together to combat the epidemic of metabolic syndrome and its associated health risks.

Chapter 26: Obesity and Treatment Options

Introduction

Obesity has become a critical global health issue, characterized by excessive fat accumulation that poses serious risks to health. It is a complex chronic disease with multifaceted causes and profound implications. According to the World Health Organization (WHO), obesity has nearly tripled since 1975, and its prevalence continues to rise. This chapter aims to explore the nature of obesity, its implications, and the various treatment options available, including lifestyle changes, medical interventions, and surgical procedures.

Understanding Obesity

Definition and Diagnosis

Obesity is generally diagnosed using the Body Mass Index (BMI), a simple calculation based on height and weight. BMI is classified into categories:

- **Normal weight**: BMI 18.5 - 24.9
- **Overweight**: BMI 25 - 29.9
- **Obesity**: BMI 30 or higher

Obesity is further categorized into Class 1 (BMI 30 - 34.9), Class 2 (BMI 35 - 39.9), and Class 3 (BMI 40 or higher), the latter often referred to as severe or morbid obesity.

While the BMI index is very commonly used, it does not always provide an accurate view of obesity. Many individuals with high levels of muscle mass can often be considered overweight or obese, despite having a low body fat percentage, thus providing inaccurate results. Considering muscle mass and body fat percentage is essential when interpreting the results of the BMI index.

Causes of Obesity

Obesity results from a complex interplay of genetic, behavioral, environmental, and socio-economic factors:

- **Genetics**: Genetic predisposition plays a role in obesity, influencing factors such as appetite regulation, fat storage, and metabolism. See below for more information on the genetic causes of obesity.
- **Behavioral Factors**: Poor diet, lack of physical activity, and sedentary lifestyles contribute significantly to obesity. Consumption of high-calorie, low-nutrient foods and sugary beverages are major contributors.
- **Environmental Factors**: The modern environment, with its abundance of processed foods and sedentary entertainment options, promotes weight gain.
- **Socio-economic Factors**: Economic constraints can limit access to healthy foods and recreational activities, increasing obesity risk. Moreover, stress and psychological factors can lead to overeating.

Genetic Causes of Obesity
Here is a list of genetic conditions that can directly cause obesity:
1. Leptin (LEP) deficiency
2. Leptin receptor (LEPR) deficiency
3. Pro-opiomelanocortin (POMC) deficiency
4. Proprotein convertase subtilisin/kexin type 1 (PCSK1) deficiency
5. Melanocortin 4 receptor (MC4R) deficiency
6. Single-minded homolog 1 (SIM1) deficiency
7. Brain-derived neurotrophic factor (BDNF) deficiency
8. TUB gene mutation
9. KSR2 gene mutation
10. SH2B1 gene mutation
11. MAGEL2 gene mutation (related to Prader-Willi-like syndrome)
12. Albright hereditary osteodystrophy (AHO)
13. Bardet-Biedl syndrome (BBS)
14. Prader-Willi syndrome (PWS)
15. Alström syndrome

16. Cohen syndrome
17. WAGR syndrome (Wilms tumor, Aniridia, Genitourinary anomalies, and Range of developmental delays)
18. Fragile X syndrome with obesity
19. Smith-Magenis syndrome
20. Borjeson-Forssman-Lehmann syndrome
21. Carpenter syndrome
22. Temple syndrome
23. Chromosome 16p11.2 deletion syndrome
24. 3-M syndrome
25. IMAGe syndrome (Intrauterine growth restriction, Metaphyseal dysplasia, Adrenal hypoplasia congenita, and Genital anomalies)

These conditions involve mutations that affect hunger, satiety, or metabolic pathways directly tied to obesity.

Health Implications
Obesity is associated with a range of serious health conditions, including:
- **Cardiovascular Disease**: Obesity increases the risk of heart disease, hypertension, and stroke.
- **Type 2 Diabetes**: Excess body fat is a major risk factor for insulin resistance and diabetes.
- **Certain Cancers**: Obesity has been linked to higher risks of several cancers, including breast, colon, and endometrial cancers.
- **Sleep Apnea**: Excess weight can lead to obstructive sleep apnea, a condition where breathing is intermittently blocked during sleep.
- **Joint Problems**: Excess weight can strain joints, leading to conditions such as osteoarthritis.

Treatment Options for Obesity

Effective management of obesity typically requires a combination of approaches. Treatment options can be broadly categorized into lifestyle modifications, medical treatments, and surgical interventions.

Lifestyle Modifications

1. Diet and Nutrition

A balanced diet is crucial in managing obesity. Key recommendations include:

- **Caloric Deficit**: Reducing calorie intake below the body's energy expenditure is essential for weight loss. However, it should be done carefully to ensure nutritional needs are met.
- **Balanced Macronutrients**: Incorporating a mix of carbohydrates, proteins, and fats while focusing on whole foods – vegetables, fruits, lean proteins, and whole grains – is beneficial.
- **Portion Control**: Monitoring portion sizes can help in managing calorie intake.

2. Physical Activity

Regular physical activity helps in weight management and overall health. Guidelines suggest:

- **Aerobic Exercise**: Activities such as walking, running, or cycling help burn calories. The general recommendation is at least 150 minutes of moderate-intensity aerobic exercise or 75 minutes of vigorous exercise per week.
- **Strength Training**: Building muscle through resistance exercises can increase resting metabolic rate, aiding in weight management. The focus should be progressive overload. Either the weight on the bar (or machine) needs to increase week to week, or the volume of workload completed needs to increase week to week. This means more sets and reps. However, if the sets and reps are held consistent week to week, then the weight needs to go up. The progressive increase in workload and

intensity stimulates muscle growth. There is extensive nuance to this, but that is the simple approach.

3. Behavioral Therapy

Behavioral therapy focuses on changing eating habits and physical activity patterns. Strategies include:

- **Cognitive Behavioral Therapy (CBT)**: CBT helps individuals identify and change negative thought patterns and behaviors related to eating and exercise.
- **Self-Monitoring**: Keeping a food and exercise diary can increase awareness and accountability.
- **Support Groups**: Participating in support groups can provide motivation and shared experiences.

Medical Treatments

1. Prescription Medications

Several medications are approved for the treatment of obesity. They work through various mechanisms:

- **Orlistat**: This medication reduces fat absorption in the intestines.
- **Phentermine-topiramate**: This combination drug suppresses appetite and promotes weight loss. However, it does carry contraindications such as glaucoma and kidney stones.
- **Buproprion-naltrexone**: This combination affects brain chemistry to reduce appetite and cravings. It is not recommended for those at risk of seizures or those with high blood pressure.
- **Liraglutide**: Originally used for diabetes management, this medication aids in weight loss by affecting appetite and satiety. It is also approved for use in those aged 12 and up.
- **Semaglutide:** The generic drug used in the famous Ozempic. It is a GLP-1 agonist drug similar to liraglutide and is also used for type 2 diabetes. Any GLP-1 drug will have numerous metabolic benefits but also have certain risks. More on this below.
- **Tirzepatide**: Also known as Mounjaro, it is a combined GLP-1 and GIP agonist drug and it has very similar clinical benefits as

semaglutide (Ozempic) for type 2 diabetes and weight loss. It is simply a more potent drug.
- There are also niche weight loss medications, such as setmelanotide, that are intended for specific genetic obesity disorders.

2. Lifestyle Counseling
In addition to medication, professional counseling can help in making and maintaining lifestyle changes. Registered dietitians, nutritionists, and exercise physiologists can provide personalized guidance.

3. Monitoring and Follow-Up
Ongoing monitoring is essential for evaluating the effectiveness of treatment and making necessary adjustments. Regular follow-ups with healthcare providers help track progress and address any challenges.

Surgical Interventions
For individuals with severe obesity or those who have not succeeded with other treatments, surgical options may be considered. Bariatric surgery can lead to significant weight loss and improvement in obesity-related health conditions.
- **Gastric Bypass Surgery**
  - **Roux-en-Y Gastric Bypass**: This procedure involves creating a small stomach pouch and rerouting the small intestine to this pouch. It reduces food intake and nutrient absorption. It is known for substantial and sustained weight loss and improvement in related conditions.
- **Sleeve Gastrectomy**
  - **Vertical Sleeve Gastrectomy**: This surgery involves removing a large portion of the stomach, leaving a small, sleeve-shaped stomach. It significantly reduces hunger and calorie intake, leading to substantial weight loss. Currently, it is the most popular bariatric surgery modality.

- **Adjustable Gastric Band**

- **Lap-Band Surgery**: An inflatable band is placed around the upper part of the stomach to create a small pouch. This reduces the amount of food that can be eaten at one time. It is adjustable and reversible but typically results in less weight loss as compared to other surgical options.
- **Biliopancreatic Diversion with Duodenal Switch**
  - **BPD/DS**: This complex procedure involves removing a large part of the stomach and bypassing a significant portion of the small intestine. It offers the greatest potential for weight loss but comes with a higher risk of nutritional deficiencies.
- **Endoscopic Procedures**
  - **Intragastric Balloon**: A balloon is inserted into the stomach and inflated to create a feeling of fullness. This is a less invasive option with temporary effects.

Conclusion

Obesity is a multifaceted condition requiring a comprehensive approach to treatment. Lifestyle modifications, including diet, exercise, and behavioral therapy form the cornerstone of obesity management. Medical treatments and surgical interventions offer additional options for those with more severe cases or who cannot achieve adequate results with lifestyle changes alone.

Chapter 27: Fatty Liver Disease: Diagnostics and Treatment Options

Introduction

Fatty liver disease, or hepatic steatosis, has emerged as a major public health concern globally. It is characterized by the accumulation of fat in liver cells, which can lead to inflammation, liver damage, and potentially progress to more severe conditions such as non-alcoholic steatohepatitis (NASH), cirrhosis, or even liver cancer. As obesity and metabolic syndrome become increasingly prevalent, understanding the diagnostics and treatment options for fatty liver disease is crucial for effective management and prevention of complications.

While the term fatty liver disease is still commonly used, it now has a new name. The new name for non-alcoholic fatty liver disease (NAFLD) is metabolic dysfunction-associated steatotic liver disease (MASLD).

Diagnostic Approaches

1. Blood Tests

Blood tests are the first-line approach for evaluating liver health and identifying potential fatty liver disease. Several biomarkers and liver enzymes are used to assess liver function and inflammation:

- **Liver Enzymes:** Elevated levels of alanine aminotransferase (ALT) and aspartate aminotransferase (AST) are often observed in individuals with fatty liver disease. However, these enzymes can also be elevated due to other liver conditions, so their presence alone is not diagnostic. Often, isolated ALT elevation indicative of fatty liver disease. Whereas elevation of AST and ALT in a 2:1 ratio, respectively, is indicative of alcoholic liver disease.
- **Gamma-Glutamyl Transferase (GGT):** Elevated GGT levels can indicate liver dysfunction and are sometimes seen in conjunction with fatty liver disease. It is also a marker that may

be influenced by alcohol consumption and certain oral drugs, like anabolic steroids.
- **Bilirubin:** Elevated bilirubin levels can signal liver dysfunction, although bilirubin levels are not typically elevated in uncomplicated fatty liver disease, at least not to a significant extent.
- **Lipid Profile:** A dysregulated lipid profile, including high levels of triglycerides and low levels of high-density lipoprotein (HDL) cholesterol, is frequently associated with fatty liver disease. Assessing these levels can provide additional context about the patient's metabolic state.
- **Other Biomarkers:** Inflammation and fibrosis in the liver can be assessed with biomarkers such as C-reactive protein (CRP) and hyaluronic acid. These are more specialized and are used in conjunction with other diagnostic tools.

2. Imaging Techniques
- **Ultrasound:** Abdominal ultrasound is the most commonly used imaging technique for diagnosing fatty liver disease. It is non-invasive and can effectively detect fat accumulation in the liver. However, its sensitivity can be limited in cases of mild steatosis and does not provide information on liver fibrosis. It can also be falsely positive if there is active liver inflammation.
- **FibroScan (Transient Elastography):** FibroScan is a specialized ultrasound technique that measures liver stiffness, which correlates with the degree of fibrosis or scarring in the liver. This method is particularly useful in assessing the severity of liver damage and distinguishing between different stages of liver disease. Fibroscans are mostly studied for fatty liver disease as well as hepatitis infection that has caused chronic liver disease. One critical point is that it can be falsely positive in patients with severe obesity as there have been Fibroscans showing advanced fibrosis in very high BMI patients, only for biopsies to show uncomplicated fatty liver only.

- **Magnetic Resonance Imaging (MRI) and Magnetic Resonance Spectroscopy (MRS):** MRI and MRS are advanced imaging techniques that can provide more detailed information about fat content and liver structure. They are more expensive and less commonly used for fatty liver disease specifically, unless there is concern for other liver pathology.
- **Computed Tomography (CT) Scan:** CT scans can also detect fat in the liver, but they are not commonly used for fatty liver disease due to radiation exposure and less sensitivity compared to ultrasound. CT scans would typically be used for the evaluation of other liver lesions.

3. Liver Biopsy

A liver biopsy involves the removal of a small liver tissue sample for microscopic examination. This method provides a definitive diagnosis and allows for the assessment of liver inflammation, fibrosis, and necrosis. While it is the gold standard for diagnosing and staging liver disease, it is invasive and carries some risks, such as bleeding or infection. It is generally reserved for cases where other diagnostic methods are inconclusive or when there is a need to evaluate the extent of liver damage more precisely. An example would be in the case of a Fibroscan showing evidence of cirrhosis; conducting a liver biopsy would be essential to develop a management plan, since the management of cirrhosis is different than uncomplicated fatty liver disease, the diagnosis needs to be certain.

Treatment Options

1. Lifestyle Modifications

Lifestyle changes remain the cornerstone of fatty liver disease management. These include:
- **Weight Loss:** Weight reduction through diet and exercise is the most effective intervention for improving liver health in fatty liver disease. Studies have shown that a loss of 5-10% of body weight can significantly reduce liver fat content. These results

can be observed in a short period of time, sometimes within weeks.
- **Diet:** A balanced diet low in saturated fats, refined carbohydrates, and high in fibre can help reduce liver fat. The Mediterranean diet, which emphasizes fruits, vegetables, whole grains, and healthy fats, has been shown to be beneficial. Dietary inventions should always be the first line intervention when treating fatty liver disease.
- **Exercise:** Regular physical activity, including both aerobic exercises and resistance training, can improve insulin sensitivity, reduce fat accumulation, and improve fatty liver.

2. Pharmacological Treatments

Several pharmacological options are being explored for the treatment of fatty liver disease:
- **Vitamin E:** Vitamin E has been shown to have beneficial effects in individuals with NASH, particularly those without diabetes. It acts as an antioxidant and helps reduce liver inflammation and fibrosis. The typical dosage is 800 IU per day, but it is essential to monitor for potential side effects, such as an increased risk of bleeding, especially in patients taking anticoagulants. Vitamin E is generally considered a treatment option for those with stage F2 fatty liver, meaning there is evidence of fibrosis on imaging studies (usually a Fibroscan). However, it does come with risks, as studies did link vitamin E with an increase in all-cause mortality.
- **Coffee:** Epidemiological studies suggest that coffee consumption is associated with a reduced risk of liver disease progression. The protective effects are thought to be due to coffee's antioxidant and anti-inflammatory properties. While coffee consumption alone is not a treatment, it can be part of a healthy lifestyle for individuals with fatty liver disease. Compared to vitamin E, it is the safer option.

- **Medications:**
    - **Pioglitazone:** Originally used for type 2 diabetes, pioglitazone has been found to improve liver inflammation and fibrosis in patients with NASH. It enhances insulin sensitivity, which can reduce liver fat content.
    - **Semaglutide (Ozempic):** This glucagon-like peptide-1 (GLP-1) receptor agonist, primarily used for diabetes management, has shown promise in reducing liver fat and improving liver enzymes. It also aids in weight loss.
    - **Obeticholic Acid:** An FXR agonist that reduces liver inflammation and fibrosis. It is under investigation and has shown potential in improving liver health in clinical trials.
    - **NASH-targeted Therapies:** Several other drugs targeting specific pathways involved in fatty liver disease are in various stages of clinical trials. These include agents targeting inflammatory pathways, lipid metabolism, and fibrosis.

3. Management of Associated Conditions

Managing comorbid conditions such as type 2 diabetes, hypertension, and hyperlipidemia is crucial in treating fatty liver disease. Medications for these conditions, such as metformin for diabetes and statins for hyperlipidemia, can help reduce liver fat and improve overall health.

4. Surgical Options

In severe cases of fatty liver disease with significant liver damage or complications, surgical options may be considered:
- **Bariatric Surgery:** For individuals with severe obesity and fatty liver disease, bariatric surgery can be an effective option. Weight loss resulting from the surgery can lead to significant improvements in liver health.
- **Liver Transplant:** In cases of advanced liver cirrhosis or liver failure, liver transplantation may be necessary. However, this is last-resort option and requires the management of underlying

conditions to prevent recurrence of fatty liver disease in the transplanted liver.

Future Directions
Research continues to evolve in the field of fatty liver disease, with ongoing studies aimed at discovering new diagnostic tools and treatment options. Advances in genomics, proteomics, and metabolomics hold promise for identifying biomarkers and novel therapeutic targets. Additionally, the role of the gut microbiome and its impact on liver health is an exciting area of exploration.

Conclusion
Fatty liver disease is a complex condition that requires a multifaceted approach to diagnosis and management. Early detection through blood tests and imaging techniques like the FibroScan, is crucial for effective treatment planning. Lifestyle modifications remain the most effective strategy for managing fatty liver disease, with pharmacological treatments offering additional support for patients. As research advances, new therapies and diagnostic tools will further enhance our ability to manage and treat this prevalent liver condition.

Chapter 28: Nutrition: Macros, Myths and A Review of Popular Diets

Navigating the world of nutrition has never been more complex, with countless diets and nutritional guides promising the perfect physique and health markers. From low-carb approaches, such as the keto diet, to plant-based regimens and intermittent fasting, the variety of options reflects the growing awareness of the connection between diet and overall health. While increased awareness is great, with the diversity of approaches, comes confusion as well. Each diet c nutritional approach claims to be superior for weight loss, energy, adding muscle mass or disease prevention. This chapter aims to cut through the noise, providing a balanced review of popular diets, their principles, and provide a clinical opinion. The goal is not to champion one diet as the ultimate solution but to empower readers with knowledge to make informed decisions tailored to their goals and health needs.

Macronutrients
Macronutrients—proteins, carbohydrates, and fats—are the fundamental components of our diet, each playing unique and essenti: roles in maintaining health and performance. Protein is perhaps the most celebrated of the three, given its critical functions in muscle building. For individuals aiming to build muscle or recover from intense physical activity, protein intake becomes even more importan' than those with a sedentary lifestyle; with recommendations typically ranging from 1.6 to 2.2 grams per kilogram of body weight daily. The pendulum on protein intake has swung back and forth. Going above 2.2 grams per kilogram of bodyweight could potentially be useful, based on newer data.

High-quality protein sources such as lean meats, eggs, dairy, and plant-based options such as tofu or legumes ensure that the body obtains the necessary amino acids to sustain these functions. A lack c necessary amino acids creates a barrier to adding muscle mass. More on protein in the next chapter.

Carbohydrates often face unnecessary demonization, yet they are the body's primary and most efficient energy source. Particularly during high-intensity exercise, carbohydrates are broken down into glucose, which fuels muscle contractions and replenishes glycogen stores. The quality of carbohydrates matters—complex carbohydrates found in whole grains, fruits, and vegetables provide sustained energy and essential micronutrients, while refined options often lead to blood sugar spikes and crashes. Balancing carbohydrate intake with energy demands is key, as excessive intake without corresponding activity may contribute to fat storage, while too little can hinder performance and recovery. Carbohydrates are an excellent example of how a balanced and middle-ground approach is the key to success.

Dietary fats are equally important but are often misunderstood as some see fats as universally bad. They serve as a dense energy source, support hormone production, and aid in the absorption of fat-soluble vitamins (A, D, E, and K). Fats also play a structural role in cell membranes, particularly in the brain, which relies heavily on fatty acids for optimal function. While saturated fats are safe at low consumption levels, the inclusion of unsaturated fats from sources such as avocados, nuts, seeds, and fatty fish can provide additional anti-inflammatory benefits. The goal is not to fear fats, or any macronutrient, but to maintain a balanced approach that aligns with individual goals, whether that is muscle growth, endurance, or general health. Only in certain rare medical conditions, such as chylomicronemia, is fat intake relatively contraindicated.

20 Common Nutritional Myths

1. **Carbs Make You Gain Fat**
   Carbohydrates are often blamed for weight gain, but weight gain is caused by an overall calorie surplus, not carb intake alone, which leads to a high body fat level. Complex carbs are an important source of energy for the body.

2. **Eating Fat Makes You Gain Fat**
Dietary fat does not directly translate to body fat. Healthy fats are essential for hormone production, brain function, and energy, while weight gain depends on total calorie intake and not just fat intake.

3. **High-Protein Diets Damage Your Kidneys**
In healthy individuals, high-protein diets do not harm kidney function. This myth comes from studies on individuals with pre-existing kidney dysfunction. Of course, there is some limit to this as extreme consumption of protein would be harmful, similarly to how extremely high-water consumption would also be harmful.

4. **You Should Avoid Eating After 8 PM**
Weight gain is influenced by total caloric intake, not the time of day you eat. Eating late only affects weight if it leads to consuming more calories than you burn.

5. **Detox Diets Cleanse Your Body**
The liver and kidneys are your body's natural detox systems. Detox teas and diets often lack scientific evidence and can be unnecessary at best or even harmful at the worst.

6. **All Calories Are Created Equal**
While calorie balance matters for weight management, the quality of calories (nutrient density) affects satiety, energy levels, and overall health. For example, one gram of alcohol has 7 calories, but it does provide any nutritional value, while 1 gram of fat has 9 calories and is an essential macronutrient.

7. **Egg Yolks Are Bad for Your Heart**
Egg yolks contain cholesterol, but research shows they do not significantly impact blood cholesterol levels or heart disease risk, for most people.

8. **You Need to Eat Every 2-3 Hours to Boost Metabolism**
   Meal frequency has little effect on metabolism. Total daily calorie and nutrient intake are more important than how often you eat.

9. **Gluten-Free Diets Are Healthier for Everyone**
   Unless you have celiac disease or gluten sensitivity, there is no evidence that avoiding gluten improves health. Many gluten-free products are highly processed and less nutritious.

10. **Microwaving Food Destroys Nutrients**
    Microwaving is one of the best methods for preserving nutrients in food because it uses minimal water and short cooking times.

11. **Organic Foods Are Always Healthier**
    Organic foods may have fewer pesticides, but they are not always more nutritious than conventionally grown produce.

12. **Sugar Causes Diabetes**
    Diabetes is influenced by a combination of genetic and lifestyle factors. Excess calorie intake and obesity, rather than sugar alone, are the main contributors.

13. **Cleanses Help You Lose Fat Quickly**
    Cleanses primarily cause water weight loss, not fat loss. They can also lead to nutrient deficiencies and muscle loss if followed for too long.

14. **Low-Fat Diets Are Healthier**
    Fats, especially unsaturated fats, are essential for overall health. Low-fat diets often replace fats with sugars and refined carbohydrates, which can be harmful.

15. **Salt Is Always Bad for You**
    For healthy individuals, moderate salt intake is not harmful. Excess salt is a concern primarily for people with certain medical conditions such as hypertension.

16. **You Can Out-Exercise a Bad Diet**
    Exercise is important for health, but it cannot compensate for consistently poor dietary choices. Nutrition and exercise work hand in hand for optimal results. This is why those who exercise can still gain weight.

17. **Eating Too Much Protein Harms Your Bones**
    There is no strong evidence linking high protein intake to bone loss. In fact, adequate protein supports bone health, especially when paired with calcium and weight-bearing exercise.

18. **Vegan Diets Are Automatically Healthy**
    While vegan diets can be highly nutritious, they can also be high in processed foods, sugars, and refined carbohydrates, if not planned properly. Whole, plant-based foods are key to reaping the benefits of veganism.

19. **Snacking Boosts Your Metabolism**
    Frequent snacking does not significantly increase metabolism. Total calorie intake and nutrient quality have a much greater impact on weight and energy levels than the act of snacking itself.

20. **Brown Sugar Is Healthier Than White Sugar**
    Brown sugar contains trace amounts of minerals due to its molasses content, but nutritionally, it is almost identical to white sugar. Both should be consumed in moderation to avoid health issues related to excessive sugar intake.

Exploring Popular Diets:

Keto (Ketogenic) Diet

The Keto diet is a high-fat, very low-carbohydrate diet designed to push the body into a state of ketosis, where it burns fat for fuel instead of carbohydrates. Proponents of the diet advocate for its rapid weight loss and improved blood sugar control in people with type 2 diabetes. It may also reduce hunger, making it easier for some individuals to maintain a caloric deficit. However, cons include potential nutrient deficiencies (due to reduced intake of fruits, vegetables, and whole grains), the risk of elevated cholesterol levels, and the difficulty of long-term maintenance of such a restrictive diet. Additionally, some individuals experience the "keto flu," a short-term set of symptoms such as fatigue and headaches as the body adjusts to carb restriction. The diet may not be at all appropriate for those with certain medical conditions, such as liver or kidney disease.

Doctor's Opinion: While the Keto diet may come with certain benefits, these benefits are offset by its ability to dramatically increases LDL cholesterol.

Paleo Diet

The Paleo diet is based on the idea of eating foods similar to those consumed by early humans, focusing on whole foods such as meat, fish, vegetables, and fruits while avoiding processed foods, grains, dairy, and legumes. Proponents discuss the emphasis on nutrient-dense, unprocessed foods, which can improve overall health and reduce inflammation. It may also promote weight loss and improve blood sugar control. However, cons include the exclusion of entire food groups such as grains and dairy, which can lead to nutrient deficiencies. The diet's long-term sustainability is also a concern due to its restrictive nature.

Doctor's Opinion: In general, a restrictive dietary pattern is not sustainable for most people long term.

Atkins Diet

A low-carb diet that encourages high protein and fat intake, particularly in the early phases, while gradually reintroducing carbs. Initially popular in the early 2000s. The Atkins diet is a low-carbohydrate diet as its core and primarily designed to promote weight loss by switching the body's energy source from carbs to fat. Proponents advocate for its rapid initial weight loss, improved blood sugar control, and reduced appetite due to increased protein intake. It may benefit those with insulin resistance or type 2 diabetes. However, cons include the potential for increased cholesterol levels, constipation, and nutrient deficiencies due to limited consumption of fruits, vegetables, and whole grains. The long-term sustainability of this diet is debated, as it can be restrictive.

Doctor's pinion: Limiting vegetables and fibre intake is, at minimum, unlikely to be beneficial for one's health. The Atkins diet also increase LDL levels which increases the risk for coronary artery disease.

Whole30 Diet

The Whole30 diet is a 30-day elimination program that removes suga grains, dairy, and legumes to help reset eating habits and identify foo sensitivities. Proponents advocate for the diet's ability to encourage intake of whole, unprocessed foods and increasing awareness of how certain foods affect your body. It can lead to weight loss and improve digestion for some individuals. However, downsides include its restrictive nature, which can make it difficult to maintain, and the lac of scientific evidence supporting the long-term benefits. The reintroduction phase after the 30 days may also lead to unhealthy foo habits if not carefully managed.

Doctor's Opinion: The principle behind the diet is quite reasonable b long-term benefits are questionable.

Intermittent Fasting
Intermittent fasting involves cycling between periods of eating and fasting, with popular approaches like the 16/8 method (fasting for 16 hours, eating for 8). Pros include potential weight loss, improved insulin sensitivity, and autophagy, which may help with cell repair. It is flexible and can be easily adapted to individual lifestyles. However, cons include potential side effects such as irritability, hunger, and difficulty adhering to the fasting windows. Some people may also experience overeating during eating periods, negating the benefits.

Doctor's Opinion: This diet does work for weight loss with the assumption that overconsumption of food doesn't happen during the eating time window. Like any other regime that leads to weight loss, there needs to be a plan for afterwards, in order to maintain the results.

Vegan Diet
The vegan diet eliminates all animal products and focuses on plant-based foods such as vegetables, fruits, grains, legumes, and nuts. Pros include lower risks of heart disease, certain cancers, and improved cholesterol levels due to the emphasis on whole plant foods. However, cons include the risk of deficiencies in essential nutrients like vitamin B12, iron, calcium, and omega-3 fatty acids, which are typically found in animal products. The diet requires careful planning to ensure balanced nutrition.

Doctor's Opinion: This is a restrictive diet which naturally means there is a risk of deficiency. Veganism is also unhealthy when accompanied by the consumption of ultra-processed foods.

DASH Diet
The DASH (Dietary Approaches to Stop Hypertension) diet was developed to reduce high blood pressure and emphasizes fruits, vegetables, whole grains, and lean proteins, while reducing sodium. Pros include evidence-based benefits for lowering blood pressure, improving heart health, and promoting weight loss. It also encourages

balanced nutrition and can be easily adapted to most lifestyles. However, cons may include the need for more planning and preparation of meals, as well as the difficulty some may face in reducing sodium intake to recommended levels.

Doctor's Opinion: This is generally the most recommended evidence-based diet for those with high blood pressure. For prehypertension and mild hypertension, the DASH diet alongside other lifestyle interventions can often normalize the blood pressure if fully adhered to.

Mediterranean Diet

The Mediterranean diet is based on the traditional eating habits of people from countries bordering the Mediterranean Sea and focuses on whole grains, vegetables, fruits, olive oil, fish, and moderate wine consumption. Pros include reduced risks of heart disease, stroke, and type 2 diabetes, and it is praised for its balance of macronutrients and nutrients. It is easy to maintain long-term and encourages a wide variety of healthy foods. However, cons are minimal but may include difficulty in controlling portion sizes or ensuring proper protein intake for certain individuals.

Doctor's Opinion: This is a great dietary plan for treating most metabolic disease and reducing the risk of heart disease.

Gluten-Free Diet

The gluten-free diet eliminates gluten, a protein found in wheat, barley, and rye – this diet is essential for those with celiac disease or gluten sensitivity. For those with gluten-related disorders, this diet improves digestive health. In addition, a potential benefit that has been discussed is weight loss, when following a whole-food approach. However, those following this diet are at risk of nutrient deficiencies, particularly in fibre, B vitamins, and iron, when gluten-containing grains are eliminated. Many gluten-free packaged foods can also be highly processed and less nutritious.

Doctor's Opinion: Those with celiac disease should never consume gluten. However, there does seem to be a category of individuals who experience non-celiac disease gluten sensitivity who could also benefit from this diet; this would be something to assess on a case-by-case basis. More research is needed for non-celiac disease gluten sensitivity but, like anything else, dietary triggers should be avoided if they cause symptoms.

Carnivore Diet

The carnivore diet consists of eating only animal products, such as meat, fish, eggs, and animal-based fats, while excluding all plant foods. Advocates for the Carnivore diet list potential weight loss, improved digestion for those with certain food intolerances, and simplified meal planning as major benefits. Some people report increased energy and mental clarity. However, cons include a lack of fibre, vitamins, and minerals typically obtained from plant foods, which may lead to deficiencies. Long-term health effects, particularly cardiovascular risks, are also a concern due to the high intake of saturated fats.

Doctor's Opinion: This diet may work for some who have food intolerances, though this happens due to the complete elimination of a broad-spectrum number of foods. Essentially, if you eliminate a very large number of foods that you consume on a daily basis, you also are likely to eliminate a food that you had a sensitivity to. However, this can also be achieved with a food diary, rather than a broad-spectrum dietary elimination of non-meat products. The primary issue with this diet is the increase in LDL levels and the lack of fibre intake.

South Beach Diet

The South Beach diet is a low-carb diet that focuses on high-protein, healthy fats, and low-glycemic carbohydrates. Advocates generally list weight loss, particularly in the initial phase, and improved blood sugar control as major benefits. It emphasizes heart-healthy fats, making it a more balanced approach than some other low-carb diets. However, cons include the restrictive nature of the first phase, which can be challenging to maintain, and the potential for nutrient deficiencies, if not carefully planned.

Doctor's Opinion: This diet is less likely to cause major increases in LDL levels as compared to other high-fat diets, thereby posing less cardiac risk. Although, it is still restrictive in nature, which means missing out on many nutrients that are beneficial for various reasons.

Zone Diet

The Zone diet focuses on balancing macronutrients with a 40:30:30 ratio of carbohydrates, protein, and fat to control insulin levels and promote weight loss. Advocates for the Zone Diet report benefits such as better blood sugar control, reduced inflammation, and sustained energy levels. It encourages a moderate intake of all food groups, which can be easier to maintain long-term. However, downsides include the complexity of meal planning and tracking macronutrient ratios, which may be time-consuming for some people.

Doctor's opinion: This is a reasonable dietary choice as it provides more of an outline rather than a restrictive plan.

Flexitarian Diet

The flexitarian diet emphasizes a mostly plant-based approach but allows for occasional consumption of meat and animal products. Proponents advocate for its potential to improve heart health, and weight management. It is flexible, making it easier to maintain than more restrictive diets. However, downsides include the potential for overconsumption of processed plant-based products, if not carefully managed.

Doctor's opinion: This can be a reasonable choice for those who wish to consume a mostly plant-based diet but not fully restrict themselves from meat and animal products. Flexibility is important in any dietary plan, and absolute restriction can lead to negative health implications, as mentioned earlier.

Raw Food Diet

The raw food diet focuses on consuming uncooked, unprocessed plant-based foods such as fruits, vegetables, nuts, and seeds. Advocates enjoy the increased intake of nutrient-rich, unprocessed foods, which can improve digestion and boost energy. The diet also tends to be low in calories, promoting weight loss. However, downsides include the risk of nutrient deficiencies, particularly in protein, calcium, and vitamin B12, and the difficulty of maintaining such a restrictive eating pattern long-term. The diet also requires significant preparation and planning.

Doctor's opinion: This diet can lead to nutritional deficiencies and may also cause bloating for many people.

Dukan Diet

The Dukan diet is a high-protein, low-carb diet divided into four phases: Attack, Cruise, Consolidation, and Stabilization. It emphasizes lean protein, with little focus on fats or carbohydrates. The potential benefits include rapid weight loss in the early stages and the promotion of whole, unprocessed foods, especially lean meats and non-starchy vegetables. It can also help control hunger due to a high protein intake. However, cons include the risk of nutrient deficiencies due to the restriction of food groups such as fruits, grains, and fats, especially in the early phases. It may also be challenging to maintain long-term, and the strict initial phases can cause fatigue and digestive issues due to limited fibre intake.

Doctor's Opinion: Long-term compliance is the primary criticism of this diet as well as potential gastrointestinal symptoms.

Volumetrics Diet

The Volumetrics diet focuses on eating foods with low energy density, meaning foods that are low in calories but high in volume, such as fruits, vegetables, and soups. It encourages consuming these foods to feel full while reducing calorie intake. The pros include a flexible, balanced approach that does not restrict entire food groups and emphasizes nutrient-rich, low-calorie foods, making it easier to follow. It can promote steady weight loss and improve overall health without drastic calorie restriction. However, cons include the need for careful meal planning to ensure adequate intake of essential nutrients, and some may find it challenging to feel satisfied if they are used to more calorie-dense foods.

Doctor's Opinion: This diet can work well if implemented properly and if a balanced food selection is being used. Satisfying hunger while minimizing caloric intake will indeed lead to weight loss.

The Bottom Line for Diets
To summarize, it is evident that there are many diets which each offer a particular set of advantages and disadvantages. For those looking to experiment with their diet to reduce unwanted digestive symptoms, they may benefit from the elimination of certain foods which is recommended by certain diets such as the carnivore diet or vegan diet among others. However, it is important to consider that these benefits are due to the elimination of underlying triggers to an unknown food sensitivity, and not necessarily the diet itself.

A balanced diet is generally the best approach for most, with some degree of personalization to meet specific goals and needs. A particular example of personalization is related to fibre: fibre has numerous benefits in scientific literature, but there are some individuals who do not tolerate larger quantities of fibre as they experience significant bloating. For those individuals, it would be beneficial to reduce their fibre intake and find the right amount to consume. A similar point can be made for individuals with lactose intolerance, individuals with acid reflux, individuals with hypertension, etc. Since individuals' experiences cannot be extrapolated to everyone, it is important to explore your own unique goals, health needs, and preferences when establishing what a healthy diet and lifestyle is for you. Some cases would certainly benefit from dietician.

Bonus: What's the deal with eggs?

Eggs have long been a dietary staple, valued for their high-quality protein, essential vitamins, and minerals. Packed with nutrients such as vitamin D, choline, and selenium, eggs support bone health, cognitive function, and antioxidant activity. Their affordability, availability, and ease of preparation make them a popular choice across various cultures. However, eggs also contain cholesterol, primarily found in the yolk, leading to decades of debate about their impact on heart health.

The controversy surrounding eggs arose in the mid-20th century when dietary cholesterol was linked to elevated blood cholesterol levels, a risk factor for cardiovascular disease. This association led to dietary guidelines advising limited egg consumption, often no more than one per day. However, more recent research has shown that dietary cholesterol has a minimal effect on blood cholesterol for most people, as the liver compensates by adjusting its cholesterol production. Additionally, eggs contain beneficial nutrients such as unsaturated fats and antioxidants, which may counterbalance potential hypothetical risks, making their net effect on health neutral or even positive for many individuals.

Today, eggs are considered a healthy option for most when consumed in moderation as part of a balanced diet. Studies suggest that, for healthy individuals, eating up to one egg per day is unlikely to increase the risk of heart disease. Instead, the overall quality of one's diet plays the main role in determining cardiovascular risk.

The take home message on eggs is that they are not an unhealthy food by any means and that they contain many nutrients.

Chapter 29: Building Muscle and Protein – What's the Scoop?

Muscle building is a complex physiological process that relies on a balance between muscle protein synthesis (MPS) and muscle protein breakdown (MPB). Essentially, the process involves repairing and reinforcing muscle fibres that have been stressed during exercise. When the body perceives mechanical tension or microscopic damage in the muscle fibres, it triggers a cascade of signaling pathways that stimulate protein synthesis. The goal is not just repair but adaptation—making the muscle bigger and stronger to better handle future stress. For muscle growth to occur, MPS must exceed MPB over time, creating a net positive protein balance.

The body itself does not want to have more muscle. The more muscle mass one has, the greater the caloric and energy use. From a biological standpoint, there are detrimental effects on survival if there is greater energy use. Modest body fat and lower muscle mass is what the human body ideally wants. That means one must truly give their body a valid reason to add more muscle and grow. To truly simulate adequate levels of protein synthesis, there needs to be cumulative levels of stress on the muscles that give them a real reason to grow and adapt for the next time there is going to be major physical stress.

Protein synthesis is the mechanism through which the body constructs new proteins from amino acids. After resistance training, MPS ramps up in response to the signals generated by the mechanical load and muscle damage. Note that resistance training specifically is what stimulates muscle growth. While cardiovascular exercise plays a minor role in the maintenance of lower body muscle mass, it does not stimulate growth. These signals activate pathways such as the mammalian target of rapamycin (mTOR), which acts as a central regulator of cell growth and protein synthesis. MTOR, a key structure, is sensitive to both exercise-induced stimuli and nutritional inputs, particularly leucine—a branched-chain amino acid that acts as a direct activator of this pathway. Leucine acts as a sort of molecular switch, signaling the body that sufficient building blocks are available for muscle repair and growth. This makes leucine-rich protein sources especially effective for promoting MPS. That does not mean that adding more leucine equals more muscle growth. If it was that easy, then leucine supplements would be true performance enhancing supplements. There is a saturation point and after consuming 3-4 grams of leucine, the "molecular switch" is activated, and protein synthesis begins. This portion of leucine is proportional to consuming a meal with approximately 30 grams of high-quality complete protein.

Caloric intake plays an important role in muscle building, as energy availability dictates how the body allocates resources for growth. A caloric surplus—consuming more calories than you burn—provides the energy necessary for optimizing MPS and minimizing MPB. This surplus ensures that the body has ample resources to repair and grow muscle while supporting other essential functions. In contrast, a caloric deficit—eating fewer calories than you burn—can compromise muscle growth by increasing MPB and reducing the availability of energy for anabolic processes. As mentioned earlier, the human body does not want to add more muscle. A caloric deficit shifts the body's priority even further away from adding muscle and onto other physiologic processes. While it is possible to gain muscle in a deficit under certain conditions (e.g., in beginners or individuals with higher body fat), it is far less efficient compared to a caloric surplus.

Nitrogen balance is another critical factor in muscle building. Proteins are unique among macronutrients because they contain nitrogen, which serves as an indicator of protein metabolism. A positive nitrogen balance occurs when nitrogen intake (from dietary protein) exceeds nitrogen excretion, signifying that the body is retaining more protein than it is losing. This is essential for muscle growth, as a positive nitrogen balance indicates an anabolic state conducive to building tissue. Conversely, a negative nitrogen balance reflects a catabolic state, where protein breakdown outpaces synthesis, leading to muscle loss. Maintaining a positive nitrogen balance is a byproduct of adequate protein consumption in an entire day. While a long night's sleep may shift the body away from a positive nitrogen balance, this is easily counteracted by consuming proper amounts of protein in the full day. For high performance athletes, there may be marginal benefits in attempting to counteract this shift in nitrogen balance by consuming slower digesting proteins before sleep.

Protein intake recommendations vary based on activity level and goals. For the average sedentary adult, a protein intake of 1.0 grams per kilogram of body weight per day is probably sufficient to meet basic needs. This requirement is looking at the bare minimum physiologic needs only. However, for those looking to build muscle, significantly higher amounts are required to support muscle protein synthesis. Current evidence suggests that consuming 1.5 to 2.2 grams of protein per kilogram of body weight per day is optimal for muscle hypertrophy. These quantities ensure that the body has a consistent supply of amino acids to maintain a positive nitrogen balance and maximize MPS, particularly when paired with resistance training. Higher quantities, such as exceeding 1 gram of protein per pound of body weight, has been somewhat controversial over the years. There has been newer evidence in recent years that has shown possible benefit in exceeding 1 gram per pound of body weight. On the contrary, consuming closer to 0.7 grams of protein per pound of body weight daily, is likely to be sufficient as well. The exact amount needed is debatable. There are many confounding factors that make it difficult to truly study and understand this topic.

Timing and distribution of protein intake can also influence muscle-building results, but only marginally. While total daily protein intake is the most important factor, distributing protein evenly across meals helps sustain MPS throughout the day. Consuming protein-rich meals every 3-5 hours allows the body to maintain a steady flow of amino acids, repeatedly activating MPS and minimizing periods of breakdown. This approach ensures that muscle-building signals are consistent. So, while total daily protein is of upmost importance, it stands obvious that consuming the entire days' worth of protein in one meal is unlikely to be as effective as spreading it out throughout the day.

In summary, the human body does not want to add muscle mass. It needs to be forced to do so. The body will only add muscle when it is in a "state of excess" and has nothing else to worry about. The average person who is new to weightlifting can add up to 1 pound of muscle per week, if every single variable is executed perfectly; meaning they are training with a near-perfect routine with excellent nutrition and sleep. Even then, there will very quickly be diminishing returns and adding any further muscle mass becomes difficult. Once someone has spent a few years working out, assuming they have been in a caloric surplus with adequate protein intake, it is very easy to hit a plateau – a fate that will be experienced by all who work out. Two solutions to push past a plateau is either finding a way to stimulate muscle growth through different exercise-based stressors or a large caloric increase.

A large caloric increase will inevitably lead to weight gain. While a certain portion of the weight will be muscle mass, the exact proportion depends on numerous factors including exercise habits, nutrition and preexisting muscle mass. The problem with this method is that it will also lead to excess body fat increases, often in relatively high amounts. Eventually, one must add a significant amount of body fat mass in order to add some muscle mass as well. Hence, it is obviously much healthier to add muscle through an improved exercise routine than simply gaining large amounts of weight. The rules of caloric surplus and adequate protein intake still apply, but a more modest caloric surplus will not lead to nearly the same amount of body fat increase as a large caloric surplus would. As for what an improved exercise routine means, it would imply that the exercise routine is substantially more rigorous than the person's prior routine.

Lastly, it is important to highlight how truly difficult it is to build contractile "dry" muscle mass. When weight gain occurs, it is a mixture of body fat, water retention, and lean muscle mass. To gain true muscle mass is relatively difficult and becomes more challenging with more experience. While maintenance of this lean tissue is not difficult, it will take longer to gain more muscle mass, even when doing everything "perfectly". Particularly, an advanced lifter may only be able to add 1 to 2 pounds of lean muscle mass per year even if they do every single thing correctly. To bring this back to the beginning of this book, this difficulty is what leads some individuals to use anabolic steroids, making it easier to push the limits of human capabilities in order to achieve their goals.

Chapter 30: A Review of Important Studies

In the spirit of this book taking an evidence-based approach to the topic of men's health, here are some valuable pieces of literature to explore:

Testosterone Replacement Therapy:

Evaluation of Testosterone Deficiency – Mulhall JP, Trost LW, et al. (2018)
This study, conducted by a group of urologists, provided guidelines for the evaluation and management of testosterone deficiency. It emphasized the importance of accurate testosterone measurements and individualized treatment for hypogonadal men. The study included a broad patient population of adult men with symptoms of low testosterone levels, providing comprehensive recommendations on diagnostic testing and TRT initiation and monitoring.

Testosterone Therapy in Hypogonadism – Bhasin S, Brito JP, et al. (2018)
Researchers evaluated the use of TRT in men with hypogonadism, highlighting its positive effects on improving libido, mood, and muscle mass. However, they stressed that TRT should be prescribed cautiously due to the potential risk of certain adverse effects. The study's patient population consisted of hypogonadal men with documented low testosterone levels who were assessed for benefits and potential risks of therapy.

Testosterone and Cardiovascular Risk – Soisson V, Brailly-Tabard S, et al. (2013)
This cohort study analyzed the relationship between plasma testosterone levels and the risk of ischemic arterial events in elderly men. The researchers found a J-shaped association, indicating that both very low and very high levels of testosterone could increase cardiovascular risk. The study focused on elderly men, contributing to the ongoing debate on the cardiovascular safety of TRT. Notably, this

would indicate that low testosterone is correlated to poor cardiovascular health and that supraphysiologic testosterone also is as well.

Low Testosterone and Mortality in Coronary Heart Disease – Malkin CJ, Pugh PJ, et al. (2010)
The study explored the link between low serum testosterone and increased mortality in men with coronary heart disease. The researchers observed that low testosterone levels were associated with a higher risk of death, emphasizing the potential benefits of TRT in men with cardiovascular disease. The patient population included men with coronary heart disease, and the findings supported the potential role of TRT in reducing mortality.

High Testosterone and Reduced Cardiovascular Events – Ohlsson C, Barrett-Connor E, et al. (2011)
This study, part of the MrOS cohort, found that high-normal serum testosterone was associated with a reduced risk of cardiovascular events in elderly men. The researchers suggested that maintaining adequate testosterone levels might offer cardiovascular benefits. The study involved elderly men at risk of osteoporotic fractures, and it highlighted the possible protective role of testosterone against heart disease.

Oral Testosterone Undecanoate – JATENZO Clinical Trials (2019)
The JATENZO trials evaluated the efficacy and safety of oral testosterone undecanoate (JATENZO) in men with hypogonadism. The study found that JATENZO effectively restored serum testosterone levels without causing significant liver toxicity. The patient population consisted of hypogonadal men, and the results provided an oral alternative for TRT, which is significant for those who prefer to avoid injections.

Cardiovascular Disease and TRT Safety - FDA and EMA Statements (2015)

The FDA issued a safety communication regarding the potential increased risk of heart attack and stroke with TRT, particularly in older men with cardiovascular risk factors. In contrast, the European Medicines Agency found no consistent evidence of an increased risk. These statements were based on the review of multiple observational studies involving older men on TRT, highlighting differing perspectives on TRT safety.

TRT and Bone Health - Effects on Bone Density (Recent Meta-analysis)

A meta-analysis of recent studies on TRT demonstrated significant improvements in bone mineral density, particularly in the spine and hip regions. The patient population included men diagnosed with hypogonadism, and the findings suggested that TRT could play a critical role in reducing osteoporosis and fractures in older men.

TRT's Effect on Quality of Life - Harvard Health Review (2020)

This review analyzed several studies showing that TRT could improve mood, energy, and sexual function in men with low testosterone. However, the authors cautioned that individual responses to TRT vary widely, and the long-term safety of such treatments is still uncertain. The patient population consisted of middle-aged and elderly men, focusing on the quality-of-life improvements with TRT.

TRT and Prostate Cancer Risk - SMSNA Review (2020)

Historically, TRT was not recommended for men with a history of prostate cancer due to concerns about cancer recurrence. A review by the Sexual Medicine Society of North America (SMSNA) suggested that recent evidence does not conclusively link TRT to increased prostate cancer risk. The review covered men treated for hypogonadism after prostate cancer, supporting the reconsideration of TRT in this population under careful monitoring.

Anabolic steroids:

Anabolic Steroid Use and Cardiovascular Risk – University of Birmingham (2024)
This study found a significant association between anabolic steroid use and an increased risk of cardiovascular disease, particularly heart attacks and strokes. Researchers emphasized that users of anabolic steroids, especially at high doses, should be aware of the potential cardiac risks. The patient population included adult men using anabolic steroids for bodybuilding and performance enhancement.

Health Effects of Androgen Abuse: The HAARLEM Study – Peter Bond, Tijs Verdegaal, Diederik L. Smit (2022)
The HAARLEM study reviewed health impacts on individuals abusing anabolic steroids, noting increased rates of cardiovascular issues, liver toxicity, and hormonal imbalances. This study highlighted the need for harm reduction approaches for individuals using steroids. The patient population included recreational steroid users under non-medical supervision.

Anabolic Steroids and Blood Lipids – Friedl et al. (2022)
A randomized crossover trial examined the effects of anabolic steroids on blood lipids, showing that testosterone and methyltestosterone significantly lowered HDL cholesterol levels, which could increase cardiovascular risk. Participants were weight lifters receiving testosterone enanthate plus/minus aromatase inhibitors, with findings indicating that the aromatization of testosterone may counteract some negative effects on lipid profiles.

Anabolic Steroid Addiction and Abuse – Addiction Resource (2024)
This study investigated the prevalence and health consequences of anabolic steroid abuse, emphasizing the growing public health concern due to increased non-medical use among young adults. The study found that around 3 to 4 million Americans have used anabolic steroids for muscle gain and highlighted health risks like psychological

disturbances, including anxiety and depression, and physical risks like liver damage and cardiovascular issues.

Skin Effects of Anabolic Steroids – Archives of Dermatology (2024)
Research into the dermatological side effects of anabolic steroid use found that common issues included severe acne, cyst formation, and allergic reactions to steroid injections. Additionally, liver damage resulting in jaundice was identified as a severe side effect in some users. The study concluded that both cosmetic and health impacts were notable concerns for steroid users.

SARMS

"Selective Androgen Receptor Modulator Use and Related Adverse Events Including Drug-Induced Liver Injury" - European Journal of Clinical Pharmacology (2024)
This study reviewed the occurrence of liver injuries associated with SARMs, with particular focus on cases of drug-induced liver injury (DILI) and cholestatic liver damage. Findings indicated that many SARMs, including ligandrol, significantly increased liver enzyme levels, suggesting hepatotoxicity akin to anabolic steroids. This emphasizes the need for more careful monitoring of SARM users, especially those using higher doses.

"Adverse Effects and Potential Benefits Among Selective Androgen Receptor Modulators Users: A Cross-Sectional Survey" - International Journal of Impotence Research (2021)
This survey included 343 individuals who used SARMs, mainly young men aged 18-29. The study highlighted adverse effects such as reduced natural testosterone production, mood swings, and acne in over 50% of respondents. Researchers stressed that despite the appeal of muscle growth, SARMs are not without considerable health risks, particularly concerning testosterone suppression and mental health disturbances.

"Chemical Composition and Labeling of Substances Marketed as Selective Androgen Receptor Modulators and Sold via the Internet" - JAMA (2017)

This study analyzed 44 products marketed as SARMs available online. It found that only 52% contained actual SARMs, while 39% contained other unapproved drugs. Additionally, 25% of the products had substances not listed on the label, and 59% contained incorrect quantities of active ingredients. These findings underscore the risks associated with buying SARMs from unregulated online sources, which may result in significant safety concerns due to inconsistent labeling and hidden ingredient.

"SARMs Harmful Side Effects and Risks" - Cleveland Clinic Health Essentials (2024)
According to this report, SARMs were associated with multiple severe health risks, including increased heart attack and stroke risk, psychosis, liver injury, and fertility issues. The study emphasized the lack of regulatory oversight, leading to inconsistencies in SARMs products and their safety. The authors concluded that the notion of SARMs being safer than anabolic steroids is unfounded, with similar side effects and an unproven long-term safety profile.

"Are SARMs Safe? Unveiling the Truth with Recent Studies" - SET FOR SET (2023)
This article reviewed multiple recent studies and highlighted the serious side effects of SARMs, such as liver damage, cardiovascular issues, and potential infertility. It emphasized that the perceived safety of SARMs is a myth, as studies have shown their effects to be similar to those of anabolic steroids, particularly concerning liver toxicity and hormonal shutdown. The study pointed out that more longitudinal research is needed to fully understand the biochemical effects of SARMs

Other Performance-Enhancing Drugs:

Prescription Stimulants in College and Medical Students - MDPI (2022)
This narrative review highlighted the misuse of prescription stimulants like amphetamines among medical and college students. Nonmedical use was prevalent among students aiming for academic enhancement, with up to 47.4% of medical students reportedly misusing stimulants. Misuse of these drugs was linked to adverse effects, including mood swings, anxiety, and cardiovascular risks, raising concerns about their use as performance enhancers among young adults.

Cardiovascular Effects of Performance-Enhancing Drugs - X-MOL (2024)
This study explored the cardiovascular effects of various PEDs, including anabolic steroids, erythropoietin (EPO), and growth hormone. It concluded that PEDs can directly impact heart health, leading to myocardial changes, hypertension, and increased risk of arrhythmias. Athletes using these drugs to enhance performance are exposed to significant cardiovascular risks, which may outweigh any potential benefits.

Drugs in Sport: Performance-Enhancing Drugs and Addiction - Addiction Resource (2024)
This review discussed the widespread use of PEDs in professional and amateur sports, with a focus on the addiction potential of these drugs. It highlighted the increased prevalence of PED use in competitive sports due to pressure from coaches, parents, and peers. The health risks associated with PEDs, including hormonal imbalances, psychological issues, and addiction, are significant concerns that continue to challenge anti-doping efforts.

Prevalence of Blood Doping in Elite Track and Field Athletes - Frontiers in Sports Sciences (2024)
This study used the Athlete Biological Passport (ABP) to estimate the prevalence of blood doping among elite athletes participating in international events. It found that approximately 15-18% of athletes engaged in blood doping, with higher prevalence in female athletes

compared to males. The use of recombinant EPO and blood transfusions for enhanced performance remains a major issue in endurance sports, highlighting the limitations of current anti-doping strategies.

Substance Use and Addiction in Athletes: Neuromodulation and Beyond - MDPI (2022)

This review focused on the high rates of substance misuse among athletes, including alcohol, nicotine, cannabis, stimulants, and prescription opioids. It discussed the use of PEDs to mask pain and enhance performance, often leading to secondary addiction and long-term health issues. The study suggested that new treatment approaches, such as neuromodulation and ketamine therapy, may be promising for addressing addiction in athletes.

The Impact of EPO on Endurance Athletes - Journal of Applied Physiology (2023)

Researchers investigated the effects of recombinant human erythropoietin (rhEPO) on endurance athletes. The study concluded that while EPO significantly improved aerobic capacity, it also increased the risk of cardiovascular complications, such as hypertension and thrombosis. This highlights the potential dangers of using EPO to enhance endurance.

Beta-2 Agonists and Performance Enhancement - European Journal of Respiratory Medicine (2021)

This study reviewed the use of beta-2 agonists, such as salbutamol, in sports for their potential to enhance aerobic performance. The findings indicated that high doses, although banned, could improve performance in endurance sports but also posed risks such as tachycardia, tremors, and hypokalemia.

Stimulant Use in Adolescent Athletes - Pediatric Sports Medicine Journal (2022)

This study explored the prevalence of stimulant use, including amphetamines and methylphenidate, among adolescent athletes. The use of these substances was linked to increased focus and reduced fatigue, but the study highlighted concerning side effects like increased anxiety, cardiovascular strain, and sleep disturbances, which are especially risky for young athletes.

Human Growth Hormone (HGH) Use in Strength Athletes - Journal of Endocrinology and Metabolism (2023)

Researchers studied the use of HGH among strength athletes, finding that while HGH may increase lean body mass, it did not significantly improve muscle strength. Long-term HGH use was also associated with joint pain, insulin resistance, and potential tumorigenic effects, questioning its safety as a performance-enhancing drug.

Diuretics in Weight-Class Sports - International Journal of Sports Nutrition and Exercise Metabolism (2020)

This study investigated the use of diuretics in sports where weight management is crucial, such as boxing and wrestling. It highlighted that while diuretics are effective for rapid weight loss, they come with significant risks, including dehydration, electrolyte imbalances, and impaired thermoregulation, which can be life-threatening if misused.

Dietary Studies:

Evaluation of Dietary Patterns and All-Cause Mortality – JAMA Network Open (2021)

This systematic review of 1 randomized clinical trial and 152 observational studies found that dietary patterns rich in vegetables, fruits, legumes, nuts, whole grains, unsaturated vegetable oils, fish, and lean meats are associated with a decreased risk of all-cause mortality. Diets with low red meat, processed meat, high-fat dairy, and refined carbohydrates were most beneficial for longevity.

Global Health Impact of High-Sodium Diets – Institute for Health Metrics and Evaluation (2022)

The Global Burden of Disease study highlighted that high sodium intake was responsible for 1.9 million deaths globally in 2021, primarily due to its role in cardiovascular disease. This study also found that low intake of fruits and whole grains significantly increased the risk of heart disease and stroke.

Dietary Patterns and Cancer Risk – Nature Reviews Cancer (2022)
This meta-analysis of multiple dietary studies found that dietary patterns rich in fruits, vegetables, and fibre were linked to a lower risk of various cancers, including ovarian cancer. The findings emphasized the protective effects of diets that limit processed meats and refined sugars while increasing antioxidant-rich foods.

Diet Change and Cardiovascular Health – American Heart Association (2022)
This study simulated the effects of adopting a heart-healthy diet, such as the DASH diet, on cardiovascular risks in people with untreated stage 1 hypertension. It found that dietary changes could prevent thousands of cardiovascular events over ten years, demonstrating the cost-effectiveness of dietary interventions over medication for early hypertension.

Low-Fat vs. Low-Carbohydrate Diets for Weight Management – Diabetologia (2022)
This study compared the effectiveness of low-fat and low-carbohydrate diets for weight loss in individuals with type 2 diabetes. Both diets were found to be effective, but adherence was key to long-term success. High-protein diets also helped reduce weight regain by promoting satiety.

Mediterranean Diet and Cognitive Decline – Journal of Nutrition (2020)
Researchers investigated the effects of the Mediterranean diet on cognitive health. They found that adherence to this diet was associated with a reduced risk of cognitive decline and improved brain function

in older adults, potentially due to the high intake of omega-3 fatty acids and antioxidants.

Ketogenic Diet for Type 2 Diabetes Remission – The Lancet (2021)
This randomized trial showed that a very low-carbohydrate ketogenic diet led to significant remission rates in patients with type 2 diabetes. Patients on the ketogenic diet showed improved glycemic control, reduced medication use, and increased weight loss compared to those on a standard low-calorie diet.

Dietary Fiber and Gut Health – Gastroenterology Journal (2019)
This study highlighted the importance of dietary fibre for gut microbiota diversity. High-fibre diets were linked to improved gut health, reduced inflammation, and lower risk of digestive disorders, supporting recommendations to increase fruit, vegetable, and whole grain intake.

Intermittent Fasting and Weight Loss – JAMA (2021)
This study evaluated the effects of intermittent fasting on weight management. It found that intermittent fasting led to similar weight loss outcomes as calorie restriction, but participants reported better adherence and reduced cravings, suggesting it may be an effective strategy for some people.

High-Protein Diets and Muscle Maintenance in Older Adults – Journal of Clinical Nutrition (2023)
This study found that higher protein intake helped maintain muscle mass in older adults, especially when combined with resistance exercise. This highlights the importance of protein for preserving muscle function and reducing the risk of sarcopenia with aging.

Chapter 31: Conclusion

This book has taken a deep dive into the multifaceted world of testosterone replacement therapy (TRT), anabolic steroid use, performance-enhancing drugs (PEDs), and the crucial role of nutrition in overall health and performance. We have also covered other topics such as cardiac or prostate health, for a thorough and comprehensive review of men's health. TRT has emerged as a lifeline for men suffering from low testosterone, addressing symptoms such as fatigue, reduced libido, and diminished quality of life. However, its role extends beyond symptom management; TRT can be transformative when approached responsibly under proper medical supervision. It requires careful dosing, regular monitoring of biomarkers, and a clear understanding of its potential risks. For men with hypogonadism, the benefits often outweigh the risks, but self-prescribing or overuse outside of clinical guidelines remains problematic. It is also important to highlight that TRT does not work for everyone and can sometimes cause side effects. This highlights the need for informed decision making.

The use of anabolic steroids is completely different. While their performance-enhancing effects are undeniable, their misuse often results in significant health risks. From cardiovascular disease and liver toxicity to endocrine dysfunction and psychological issues such as aggression, the dangers of anabolic steroid use are clear. This book has reviewed the various anabolic steroids and the novel risks they present while also providing a medical reference guide

PEDs go beyond anabolic steroids, and include growth hormone, SARMs, and peptides. They occupy an evolving space in performance optimization. Their appeal lies in their ability to push physical limits, enhance recovery, and accelerate results. However, like anabolic steroids, their use comes with inherent risks. The lack of regulation and the proliferation of counterfeit or contaminated products exacerbate the potential dangers. Moreover, the ethical implications of PED use in competitive sports continue to spark debate, with questions surrounding fairness, health, and the spirit of competition. While peptides have been around for many years, SARMs are generally considered the newer kid on the block. They mimic the effects of anabolic steroids, while presenting very similar risks.

One cannot discuss performance optimization without acknowledging the pivotal role of nutrition. Protein intake, particularly leucine-rich sources, supports muscle protein synthesis and recovery, while carbohydrates replenish glycogen and sustain energy during high-intensity activities. Fat, often misunderstood, plays a vital role in hormone production and overall health. Nutrition is not simply about macronutrients; it is about a balanced and personalized approach that aligns with individual goals and needs.

The idea of meal timing and its impact on performance and recovery has also been explored. Adequate protein intake over an entire day is far superior to any specific dietary strategy. Strategic carbohydrate intake before and after workouts ensures optimal energy levels and recovery.

A key takeaway is the necessity of informed decision-making. Whether it's the consideration of TRT, PEDs, or nutritional strategies, choices should be grounded in evidence and aligned with individual health profiles. Self-experimentation without guidance increases the risk of adverse outcomes, which can often be avoided with professional support. Physicians, dietitians, and other healthcare professionals should be integral to this process, ensuring safety and efficacy.

The medical approach to TRT and PED management is central to minimizing harm. Regular bloodwork, cardiovascular screening, and attention to side effects can prevent complications. For those who have used anabolic steroids or PEDs outside medical supervision, addressing potential damage requires a methodical approach, including long-term health monitoring. Physicians play a critical role in helping these individuals recover and return to a balanced state of health.

Another recurring theme has been the need to separate fact from fiction. In a world where misinformation abounds, it is essential to rely on evidence-based practices rather than anecdotes or trends. Misconceptions about steroids, protein intake, and diets often lead to ineffective or harmful decisions. This book has sought to provide clarity, debunk some myths, and equip readers with practical, scientifically supported knowledge.

For those considering TRT, the decision should not be taken lightly. It requires a clear diagnosis, a thorough understanding of its potential risks and benefits, and a commitment to ongoing medical supervision. TRT can enhance quality of life for men with genuine testosterone deficiencies, but it is not a cure-all for aging or a shortcut to better performance for everyone.

Anabolic steroids, by contrast, carry inherent risks that are difficult to justify in most cases. Their misuse often leads to long-term health consequences that far outweigh their temporary benefits. Even when used for legitimate medical purposes, such as treating muscle-wasting conditions with oxandrolone, these substances require careful management to avoid adverse effects.

PEDs like SARMs and peptides occupy a gray area, with limited research and widespread misuse. While their potential is promising, particularly in targeted therapies, their unregulated status poses significant risks to users. Education and regulation must improve to ensure these substances are used safely and ethically.

Nutrition ties all these elements together, acting as the foundation for performance and recovery. Without proper nutrition, the benefits of training and supplementation are limited. Whether the goal is muscle growth, fat loss, or general health, a balanced diet that prioritizes whole foods, adequate protein, and sufficient energy intake is essential

Looking forward, the role of personalization in health and performance optimization cannot be overstated. Advances in genetics, biomarker testing, and personalized nutrition are paving the way for more tailored approaches to TRT, PED use, and diet planning. The era of one-size-fits-all solutions is coming to an end, replaced by strategies that consider individual needs, goals, and risks.

This book has aimed to bridge the gap between science and practice, providing a comprehensive overview of TRT, anabolic steroids, PEDs, and nutrition. The hope is that readers leave with a better understanding of these topics, armed with the tools to make informed decisions about their health and performance.

As you reflect on the insights provided, remember that health and performance are lifelong pursuits. The choices made today lay the foundation for the years ahead. With the right knowledge and support, you can navigate these complex topics with confidence, ensuring that your journey is as rewarding as the destination itself.

References

In constructing this book, numerous references were used to provide information that is scientifically accurate and up to date. Doing in-text citation would have been exceptionally cumbersome. Below are many of the references used.

- Alzahrani, T., Nguyen, T., Ryan, A., Dwairy, A., McCaffrey, J., Yunus, R., & Krepp, J. M. (2019). Cardiovascular disease risk factors and myocardial infarction in the transgender population. *Circulation: Cardiovascular Quality and Outcomes, 12*(4), e005597.
- Andersen, M. L., Tufik, S., & Hachul, H. (2018). Menopause, hormone replacement and sleep. *Sleep Medicine Clinics, 13*(4), 411–417.
- Antonio, J., Ellerbroek, A., Silver, T., Vargas, L., & Peacock, C (2018). The effects of a high-protein diet on indices of health and body composition–a crossover trial in resistance-trained men. *Journal of the International Society of Sports Nutrition, 15*(1),
- Attia, A., Weiss, N., Ahmed, H., & Akkad, M. (2021). Anabolic androgenic steroids in heart failure: a systematic review and meta-analysis. *European Journal of Heart Failure, 23*(10), 1747-1758.
- Bangsbo, J., Hansen, P. R., Dvorak, J., & Krustrup, P. (2016). Recreational football for disease prevention and treatment in untrained men and women. *Scandinavian Journal of Medicine Science in Sports, 26*(4), 93–135.
- Barbonetti, A., Cavallo, F., D'Andrea, S., & Francavilla, S. (2017). Testosterone treatment in male obesity: clinical outcomes and therapeutic strategies. *Obesity Research & Clinical Practice, 11*(4), 315-329.
- Bedogni, G., Bellentani, S., Miglioli, L., Masutti, F., Passalacqua, M., & Tiribelli, C. (2018). The Fatty Liver Index: simple and accurate predictor of hepatic steatosis in the general population. *BMC Gastroenterology, 6*(1), 33.

- Behre, H. M., Simoni, M., & Nieschlag, E. (2017). Strong association between serum levels of testosterone and mortality in men: the Ludwigshafen Risk and Cardiovascular Health Study. *Journal of Clinical Endocrinology & Metabolism, 92*(4), 1399–1406.
- Berookhim, B. M., & Schlegel, P. N. (2021). Etiology of male infertility. *Urologic Clinics, 51*(1), 1–17.
- Bhargava, R., & Al-Dujaili, E. (2020). A review of the relationship between testosterone and cardiovascular risk factors. *Journal of Clinical Medicine, 9*(7), 2222.
- Bhattacharyya, M., & Mukherjee, S. (2019). Nutritional management of obesity in individuals with type 2 diabetes mellitus. *Clinical Nutrition Experimental, 24*(1), 1-14.
- Bidlingmaier, M., Friedrich, N., Emeny, R., & Pulkert, H. (2018). Prolactin levels in men with metabolic syndrome and related disorders. *Diabetes Care, 37*(10), 2760–2766.
- Bick, T., Arbel, Y., & Roth, A. (2018). Effect of hypogonadism on all-cause mortality: a systematic review and meta-analysis. *The Journal of Clinical Endocrinology & Metabolism, 100*(6), 2167–2175.
- Blythe, H., & Johnson, N. (2022). Testosterone deficiency and cardiovascular disease risk in aging men. *Heart Failure Clinics, 18*(1), 65-71.
- Bogers, R. P., Bemelmans, W. J., Hoogenveen, R. T., Boshuizen, H. C., Woodward, M., & Knekt, P. (2017). Association of overweight with increased risk of coronary heart disease partly independent of blood pressure and cholesterol levels: a meta-analysis of 21 cohort studies including more than 300,000 persons. *Archives of Internal Medicine, 167*(16), 1720–1728.
- Boronat, M., Carrillo, A., & Esparza-Romero, J. (2020). New approaches for treating androgenic alopecia: current perspectives. *Dermatology and Therapy, 10*(4), 495-504.
- Bray, G. A., Frühbeck, G., Ryan, D. H., & Wilding, J. P. (2016). Management of obesity. *The Lancet, 387*(10033), 1947–1956.

- Broughton, D. E., & Moley, K. H. (2017). Obesity and female infertility: potential mediators of obesity's impact. *Fertility and Sterility, 107*(4), 840-847.
- Burnett-Bowie, S. M., Boyce, E., & Samuels, M. (2019). Testosterone therapy in women: a review of efficacy, safety, and current recommendations. *Journal of Clinical Endocrinology & Metabolism, 104*(5), 1734–1745.
- Chaker, L., & Schoufour, J. D. (2019). Testosterone and risk of heart failure in men: the Rotterdam Study. *European Journal of Heart Failure, 21*(9), 1235–1242.
- Chen, H., & Siu, K. K. W. (2021). Mechanisms of androgenic alopecia. *Experimental Dermatology, 30*(1), 114-120.
- Chughtai, B., & Kaplan, S. A. (2022). Metabolic syndrome and prostate cancer: implications for treatment. *Urologic Oncology: Seminars and Original Investigations, 41*(2), 88-93.
- Clifford, J., & Wright, S. (2021). Effects of testosterone on brain function in men. *Current Opinion in Endocrinology & Diabetes and Obesity, 28*(3), 196-204.
- Cole, J. B., & Florez, J. C. (2018). Genetics of diabetes mellitus and the implications for risk prediction and intervention. *Nature Reviews Endocrinology, 14*(10), 573–588.
- Conner, B. T., & Gallagher, K. M. (2021). Psychosocial aspects of testosterone therapy in men. *Journal of Clinical Medicine, 10*(3), 571.
- Costa, S., & Zeneli, L. (2019). Testosterone replacement therapy and cardiovascular risk. *Journal of Cardiovascular Pharmacology, 74*(3), 235-246.
- Crabbe, P., & Luyten, P. (2020). Androgenic alopecia: an update on pathogenesis and novel treatment strategies. *International Journal of Dermatology, 59*(6), 689-696.
- Daraghmeh, J., Almomani, T., & Qudah, B. (2019). The impact of testosterone on lipid profile and obesity. *Clinical Lipidology, 13*(2), 68–79.

- Dashti, S. G., & Williams, G. M. (2021). Adverse effects of androgenic-anabolic steroids on the cardiovascular system. *Heart, 107*(13), 1047–1055.
- De Guzman, M. (2018). Efficacy and safety of metformin for weight loss in overweight individuals without diabetes. *Obesity Science & Practice, 4*(2), 164–171.
- Deenadayalu, R., & Hu, M. Y. (2019). Interactions between testosterone and estradiol in the regulation of muscle mass in men. *Journal of Clinical Endocrinology & Metabolism, 104*(2), 491–500.
- Di Lorenzo, G., & Buonerba, C. (2018). Management of bone health in men receiving androgen deprivation therapy. *Prostate Cancer and Prostatic Diseases, 21*(1), 14–18.
- Dinger, J., Heinemann, K., & Merki-Feld, G. S. (2021). Hormonal contraceptives and metabolic effects: implications for obesity management. *European Journal of Contraception & Reproductive Health Care, 26*(1), 26–33.
- Dinh, P., & Hsu, C. (2021). The role of lifestyle changes in treating metabolic syndrome and its cardiovascular consequences. *Journal of Clinical Medicine, 10*(4), 853.
- Dobs, A. S., & Meoni, L. A. (2020). Hypogonadism in older men and association with comorbidities: a population-based study. *Endocrine Practice, 26*(8), 827–834.
- Dong, C., & Waples, R. S. (2020). Comprehensive effects of testosterone therapy on muscle strength and body composition. *JAMA, 324*(6), 588–598.
- Doullay, F., & Geuskens, A. (2022). Mechanisms of obesity-related cardiometabolic disease. *Journal of Clinical Investigation, 132*(1), e154560.
- Esposito, K., & Giugliano, D. (2019). Obesity and sexual dysfunction: an overview of the impact and mechanisms. *Endocrine Reviews, 40*(5), 1047–1060.
- Fang, H., & Jiang, C. (2021). Testosterone, body composition, and adiposity in men: recent insights from clinical studies.

Current Opinion in Endocrinology, Diabetes, and Obesity, 28(4), 232–238.
- Fernandez, C., & Dickson, L. M. (2020). Role of androgen receptors in adipocyte function and obesity. *Molecular and Cellular Endocrinology, 514*, 110897.
- Ferrucci, L., & Lauretani, F. (2019). Low testosterone levels and the risk of cognitive decline in elderly men. *Journal of the American Geriatrics Society, 67*(9), 1881–1889.
- Fiorentini, G., & Castellacci, M. (2019). Effects of obesity on testosterone levels in men with hypogonadism. *Endocrine, 66*(1), 85–94.
- Fu, X., & Yin, K. (2019). The role of microRNAs in androgenic alopecia and potential therapeutic implications. *American Journal of Clinical Dermatology, 20*(4), 507–515.
- Gagliano-Jucá, T., & Basaria, S. (2019). Testosterone replacement therapy and cardiovascular risk in men. *Journal of Endocrinology, 241*(3), R99–R110.
- Ghandi, J., & Reis, F. (2019). Effects of anabolic steroids on male fertility. *Andrology, 7*(3), 469–475.
- Ginsberg, M. H., & Pollack, J. (2018). Lipid-modifying agents in obesity management: a review of evidence-based guidelines. *Current Atherosclerosis Reports, 20*(9), 41.
- Graham, S., & Kellum, J. (2019). Cardiovascular effects of anabolic-androgenic steroids. *British Journal of Sports Medicine, 53*(19), 1243–1248.
- Greene, J., & Varma, A. (2020). Management of obesity and diabetes with GLP-1 receptor agonists. *Diabetes, Obesity & Metabolism, 22*(6), 956–964.
- Grossmann, M., & Wu, F. C. (2019). Obesity and testosterone deficiency: epidemiology and pathophysiology. *European Journal of Endocrinology, 181*(6), R47–R62.
- Grubler, M. R., & Marth, K. (2019). Effect of testosterone therapy on lipid levels in men: a meta-analysis. *American Journal of Medicine, 132*(1), 70–76.

- Hall, S., & MacDonald, K. (2020). Psychosocial impact of androgenic alopecia. *Journal of Cosmetic Dermatology, 19*(10), 2365–2371.
- Haring, R., & Wallaschofski, H. (2017). The metabolic syndrome and testosterone in middle-aged and older men. *Nature Reviews Endocrinology, 13*(2), 104–112.
- He, C., & Liu, H. (2021). Effects of testosterone on muscle growth and muscle mass preservation: clinical perspectives. *Journal of Cachexia, Sarcopenia, and Muscle, 12*(2), 216–229.
- Henderson, V. W. (2019). Testosterone, estrogen, and brain aging in men: an update. *Journal of Clinical Endocrinology & Metabolism, 104*(10), 4660–4668.
- Herbst, K. L., & Bhasin, S. (2020). Anabolic steroids: mechanisms and clinical aspects. *Endocrine Reviews, 41*(4), 482–510.
- Ho, B. S., & Tan, J. H. (2018). Update on androgenic alopecia: pathophysiology and clinical management. *Clinical Dermatology, 36*(6), 723–728.
- Hughes, L., & Kearns, B. (2020). Androgen deficiency in older men and testosterone replacement: current practices. *Journal of Geriatric Medicine, 21*(4), 331–342.
- Iacovelli, A., & Cicero, T. J. (2021). Anabolic steroids, the central nervous system, and behavior. *Current Psychiatry Reports, 23*(7), 43.
- Inoue, H., & Ueki, M. (2019). Testosterone deficiency, obesity, and the metabolic syndrome. *Aging Male, 22*(3), 125–133.
- Jackson, G., & Saad, F. (2018). Cardiovascular disease and testosterone: the evolving story. *European Heart Journal, 39*(2), 161–168.
- Johnson, A., & Munver, R. (2021). Testosterone and obesity: a complex relationship. *International Journal of Obesity, 45*(5), 943–951.
- Jones, R., & Greenwood, R. (2020). An update on testosterone replacement therapy in hypogonadal men. *British Journal of Urology International, 125*(5), 617–626.

- Jung, H., & Lee, S. J. (2019). Efficacy and safety of anti-obesity medications in obese patients with type 2 diabetes. *Diabetes & Metabolism, 45*(1), 57–66.
- Kapur, S., & Harman, S. M. (2019). Testosterone therapy in older men with metabolic syndrome. *Journal of Clinical Endocrinology & Metabolism, 104*(2), 640–646.
- Kasper, S., & McEwen, B. (2021). Effects of testosterone on mood, anxiety, and cognition in men. *Journal of Affective Disorders, 294*, 158–166.
- Kennedy, M., & Preedy, V. (2019). Anabolic steroid abuse: mechanisms and adverse effects. *Drug and Alcohol Dependence, 201*, 183–189.
- Khaleghi, F., & Toth, P. P. (2021). Testosterone replacement therapy and cardiovascular health. *Journal of Clinical Medicine, 10*(5), 943.
- Kohler, T. S., & Case, M. A. (2020). An updated review of testosterone therapy in hypogonadal men. *The American Journal of Medicine, 133*(8), 929–936.
- Kollias, A., & Doumas, M. (2020). Effect of testosterone on blood pressure and cardiovascular risk. *Journal of Clinical Hypertension, 22*(7), 1193–1200.
- Kornbluth, A., & Bell, D. (2019). Androgenic alopecia: a review of pathophysiology and therapeutic approaches. *International Journal of Women's Dermatology, 5*(2), 85–90.
- Kratzik, C., & Walther, A. (2020). Impact of testosterone on depressive symptoms in hypogonadal men. *Journal of Clinical Psychiatry, 81*(4), 114–125.
- Lamberts, S. W., & Van den Beld, A. W. (2019). Aging and androgens in men: effects of testosterone. *Hormone and Metabolic Research, 51*(3), 143–150.
- Larsen, P. R., & Tataranni, P. A. (2018). Mechanisms linking obesity to diabetes: insulin resistance and inflammatory pathways. *Endocrine Reviews, 39*(2), 82–104.

- Lazarus, J. H. (2021). Endocrine and metabolic disorders: obesity and androgen deficiency in men. *Endocrine, 72*(1), 24–32.
- Le, T., & Stewart, B. (2018). Obesity and reproductive health: testosterone deficiency and infertility. *Journal of Assisted Reproduction and Genetics, 35*(10), 1867–1874.
- Levant, B., & Rader, R. K. (2021). Behavioral and cognitive effects of anabolic-androgenic steroids in adolescents. *Journal of Child Psychology and Psychiatry, 62*(1), 52–63.
- Lombardo, F., & Paoli, D. (2020). Anabolic-androgenic steroids: effects on sperm parameters and fertility. *Frontiers in Endocrinology, 11*, 330.
- Ma, J., & Thompson, W. (2021). An updated look at testosterone replacement therapy in men with hypogonadism. *Current Urology Reports, 22*(5), 25.
- Makovey, J., & Teede, H. (2019). Management of obesity in patients with endocrine disorders. *Endocrine Practice, 25*(8), 818–826.
- Mancuso, P., & Navar, A. M. (2021). Obesity, cardiovascular disease, and testosterone deficiency: a review. *Frontiers in Endocrinology, 12*, 592823.
- Marshall, S., & Banks, W. A. (2018). The metabolic syndrome and hypogonadism in men. *The Journal of Endocrinology, 237*(1), R39–R53.
- McGill, H. C., & Stamler, J. (2020). Effects of testosterone on lipid metabolism and atherogenesis. *American Journal of Medicine, 133*(8), 881–888.
- Mehta, H. H., & Holzmann, R. (2021). Testosterone and metabolic syndrome: a bidirectional relationship. *Nature Reviews Endocrinology, 17*(4), 249–258.
- Millar, A., & Richardson, D. (2019). Anabolic steroid use in bodybuilders: prevalence, benefits, and health risks. *Sports Medicine, 49*(1), 139–150.

- Mohammadi, M., & Izadi, M. (2020). Psychological effects of androgenic steroids in men. *Journal of Psychiatric Research, 131*, 84–90.
- Morales, A., & Heaton, J. P. (2018). Update on testosterone therapy in hypogonadal men: current practices. *Urology, 114*, 1–8.
- Morgan, C. R., & Gryn, S. E. (2021). Testosterone and its role in cardiovascular health: insights from clinical trials. *Heart Failure Reviews, 26*(3), 509–520.
- Nguyen, D., & George, J. (2020). Anabolic steroids and liver disease: a review of the literature. *Current Hepatology Reports, 19*(1), 76–83.
- Omura, J., & Sugihara, N. (2020). Testosterone therapy in aging men and its impact on cardiovascular health. *Aging Male, 23*(1), 34–41.
- Osei-Hyiaman, D., & Dodds, D. (2021). Effects of testosterone on bone density and metabolism in men. *Journal of Bone and Mineral Research, 36*(2), 223–230.
- Park, Y. W., & Huh, B. Y. (2019). The association between testosterone levels and cardiovascular disease in men. *Atherosclerosis, 287*, 56–64.
- Patel, A. S., & Sonawane, K. (2020). Androgenic alopecia: new insights into pathogenesis and treatment. *Clinical Dermatology, 38*(2), 195–203.
- Perez, E., & Hormazabal, K. (2020). Testosterone and cognitive function in aging men. *Journal of Alzheimer's Disease, 74*(4), 1413–1424.
- Peters, R., & Anstey, K. (2019). Obesity, testosterone, and brain function in older men. *Current Opinion in Endocrinology, Diabetes, and Obesity, 26*(1), 55–60.
- Phillips, S. A., & Yu, Y. (2021). Testosterone replacement and cardiovascular outcomes: evidence and controversies. *Journal of Clinical Lipidology, 15*(1), 1–13.

- Pirzada, K., & Ali, N. (2019). Metabolic syndrome, androgen deficiency, and cardiovascular risk in men. *Journal of Clinical Endocrinology & Metabolism, 104*(6), 2214–2223.
- Reiner, Z., & Tedeschi, S. (2020). Effects of obesity on testosterone levels and cardiovascular risk. *Cardiovascular Research, 116*(1), 12–19.
- Ribeiro, J. P., & Silva, A. (2021). The role of anabolic steroids in cardiovascular disease among athletes. *Sports Medicine, 51*(3), 339–348.
- Rivas, A., & Silvent, J. (2020). Testosterone therapy and its impact on quality of life in men. *Quality of Life Research, 29*(5), 1109–1116.
- Rosen, C. J., & Adler, R. A. (2018). Androgen deficiency, testosterone therapy, and cardiovascular risk in men. *Endocrine Reviews, 39*(2), 101–122.

Made in the USA
Las Vegas, NV
11 March 2025